"This volume is a v [illegible] ical and scientific study of delusion. Its ch [illegible] researchers in the study of delusion, and they cover a w [illegible] opics including the ones that have been largely underexplored, such as the historical or normative issues on delusion."

Kengo Miyazono, *Hokkaido University, Japan*

THE PHILOSOPHY AND PSYCHOLOGY OF DELUSIONS

This book presents new philosophical work on delusions and their impact on everyday human behavior. It explores a cluster of related topics at the intersection of philosophy of mind and psychiatry, while also charting the historical development of work on delusions.

Within psychiatry, there are several disputes about the nature and origin of delusions. Whereas some authors see only an abnormal phenomenon that needs to be treated by psychological or pharmacological means, others hold that delusions can be psychologically adaptive and even have epistemic benefits. This book brings together an interdisciplinary group of contributors to build consensus around what delusions are and how they impact the human mind. Part 1 provides readers with an informed historical discussion of delusions and carefully examines the contemporary impact of these historical perspectives. Part 2 analyzes the impact of contemporary views of delusions on the mental and emotional life of human agents. Finally, Part 3 explores the normative frameworks of delusions and analyzes the impact of some of their behavioral consequences on the daily life of subjects and their caregivers.

The Philosophy and Psychology of Delusions is essential reading for researchers and graduate students working at the intersection of philosophy, psychiatry, and psychology.

Ana Falcato holds a PhD in Philosophy from the NOVA/FCSH, Lisbon, Portugal. Between 2013 and 2015, she was a Humboldt Research Fellow at the Johannes-Gutenberg University and the University of Oxford. Her work has appeared in *Studies in the Novel, Hypatia: A Journal of Feminist Philosophy, Kant-Studien, Wittgenstein-Studien, Daimon: Revista International de Filosofía* and the *Deutsche Zeitschrift für Philosophie*. She published *Philosophy in the Condition of Modernism* in 2018 and *Phenomenological Approaches to Intersubjectivity and Values* in 2019 (co-edited with Luís Aguiar de Sousa). In 2021 appeared her edited collection *The Politics of Emotional Shockwaves*. Ana is Assistant Researcher at

NOVA/FCSH, where she conducts a project about the novelistic and critical work of J.M. Coetzee.

Jorge Gonçalves is a Post-doctoral research fellow in Philosophy at Instituto de Filosofia da Nova (IFILNOVA), Universidade Nova de Lisboa, where he works on Philosophy of Psychiatry, Consciousness and Self-Studies, and Philosophy of Psychology. He graduated first in Psychology (1988) and afterwards in Philosophy (1997), both in Lisbon. He has a master's degree in Philosophy (2002) and a PhD (2007) in Philosophy ("Consciousness and Natural Order"). Between 1988 and 1999, he worked as a clinical psychologist (educational, learning disabilities and chronic mental illness). Gonçalves's current research is on topics in Philosophy of Psychiatry, with a special focus on the concept of mental illness, the mind-body problem and psychiatry, theories of delusion, and the problem of the unconscious. He is the author of several papers and editor of three books. Jorge was PI of the funded project 'Cognitive Foundations of the Self', sponsored by the Portuguese Foundation for Science and Technology (FCT) between 2009 and 2012.

Routledge Studies in Contemporary Philosophy

A Plea for Plausibility
Toward a Comparative Decision Theory
John R. Welch

Living with the Dead
On Death, the Dead, and Immortality
J. Jeremy Wisnewski

Free Will's Value
Criminal Justice, Pride, and Love
John Lemos

Emotional Self-Knowledge
Edited by Alba Montes Sánchez and Alessandro Salice

Global Justice and Recognition Theory
Dignifying the World's Poor
Monica Mookherjee

The Mind-Body Problem and Metaphysics
An Argument from Consciousness to Mental Substance
Ralph Stefan Weir

The Philosophy and Psychology of Delusions
Historical and Contemporary Perspectives
Edited by Ana Falcato and Jorge Gonçalves

For more information about this series, please visit: https://www.routledge.com/Routledge-Studies-in-Contemporary-Philosophy/book-series/SE0720

The Philosophy and Psychology of Delusions

Historical and Contemporary Perspectives

Edited by Ana Falcato and Jorge Gonçalves

Routledge
Taylor & Francis Group
NEW YORK AND LONDON

First published 2024
by Routledge
605 Third Avenue, New York, NY 10158

and by Routledge
4 Park Square, Milton Park, Abingdon, Oxon, OX14 4RN

Routledge is an imprint of the Taylor & Francis Group, an informa business

ISBN: 978-1-032-26591-9 (hbk)
ISBN: 978-1-032-26592-6 (pbk)
ISBN: 978-1-003-28899-2 (ebk)

DOI: 10.4324/9781003288992

Typeset in Sabon
by SPi Technologies India Pvt Ltd (Straive)

Contents

Contributors

Filipe Arantes-Gonçalves is a PhD Student at the Doctoral Program in Medicine of the Faculty of Medicine – University of Porto. He is psychiatrist by the Portuguese Medical Association and psychoanalyst by the Portuguese Association for Psychoanalysis and Psychoanalytic Psychotherapy.

Rick Bellaar holds a MSc in Logic from the University of Amsterdam, the Netherlands. In 2021 he was awarded the second prize of the biannual Van Helsdingen competition of the Dutch foundation for Philosophy and Psychiatry. His research interests include Wittgenstein and conceptual issues in psychiatry. He is currently enrolled as an external PhD candidate in Psychology under supervision of Dr. Jasper Feyaerts at the Department of Psychoanalysis and Clinical Consulting at Ghent University.

Lisa Bortolotti is Professor of Philosophy at the University of Birmingham, UK. She works in the philosophy of the cognitive sciences and has a special interest in belief, irrationality, and mental health.

Jasper Feyaerts holds a PhD in Clinical Psychology from Ghent University, Belgium. Between 2018 and 2021, he was an FWO postdoctoral research fellow at the Department of Psychoanalysis & Clinical Consulting at Ghent University and the Center for Contextual Psychiatry at KU Leuven. His research interests include phenomenological research on delusions and psychosis onset in schizophrenia spectrum disorders and conceptual research on philosophical issues in psychiatry. His work has appeared in *Lancet Psychiatry*, *Philosophy, Psychiatry & Psychology* and *Psychosis*. He is currently an Assistant Professor at the Department of Psychoanalysis & Clinical Consulting at Ghent University, where he pursues phenomenological and philosophical research on psychosis.

Shaun Gallagher is the Lillian and Morie Moss Professor of Excellence in Philosophy at the University of Memphis. Secondary appointments: Professorial Fellow in the Faculty of Law, Humanities and the Arts, University of Wollongong (Australia), and Honorary Professor of Health Sciences, Tromsø University, The Arctic University of Norway. He holds the Anneliese Maier Research Award (2012–2018) from the Humboldt Foundation.

Philip Gerrans is full-time professor of Philosophy at the University of Adelaide, Australia. His main research interest is the use of psychological disorder to study the mind. He has written on developmental disorders (autism and Williams syndrome), cognitive neuropsychiatry, on moral psychopathologies (such as psychopathology) and the emotions as well as a large monograph and associated series of papers on delusion and disorders of rationality. Gerrans is an Associate of the Swiss Centre for Affective Sciences, where he collaborates with philosophers, psychologists and neuroscientists. He is now completing a project on the relationship between emotional processing and self-representation with an emphasis on psychiatric disorders. Together with Chris Letheby, Gerrans is leading a project on philosophical issues raised by the nature of psychedelic experience. In all these cases his research focus is on the role of computational models linking experience to neural processing.

Luigi Grassi, MD, is Professor and Chair of Psychiatry, Chair of the Department of Biomedical and Specialty Surgical Sciences of the University of Ferrara, Italy, and Head of the University Unit of Hospital Psychiatry, S. Anna Hospital and Local Health Agency in Ferrara, Italy. He is author of about 200 scientific papers, chapters of books and books. He has been the President of the International Psycho-Oncology Society (IPOS) (2006–2008) and the Italian Society of Psycho-Oncology (SIPO) (2003–2011). He is currently Chair of the IPOS Federation of Psycho-Oncology Societies and the World Psychiatric Association – Section on Psycho-Oncology & Palliative Care. Dr. Grassi's clinical and research interests are in the area of psycho-oncology, consultation-liaison psychiatry and psychosomatic medicine, and psychosocial and psychiatry rehabilitation.

Pablo López-Silva, PhD, is Professor of Psychology at the Universidad de Valparaíso School of Psychology, Chile; Research Professor at the Universidad de Valparaíso Institute of Philosophy, Chile, and Young Research Fellow at the ANID Millennium Institute for Research in Depression and Personality (MIDAP). He works at the interface of psychopathology, empirically informed philosophy of mind, and phenomenology. He is currently leading a four-year FONDECYT project titled 'The Architecture of

Delusions' funded by the Government of Chile's National Agency for Research and Development (ANID). His work has been published in English and Spanish in journals such as *Schizophrenia Research*, *Review of Philosophy & Psychology*, *Psychiatric Quarterly*, *Frontiers in Psychiatry*, *Crítica*, *Tópicos*, among others.

Ashleigh Morales is a PhD student and researcher in philosophy at the University of Memphis, where she conducts work under the supervision of Professor Gallagher.

Georg Northoff holds the Canada Research Chair in Mind, Brain Imaging and Neuroethics, and the ELJB-CIHR Michael Smith Chair in Neurosciences and Mental Health, whose research unit he coordinates. He holds degrees in both philosophy and psychiatry.

Jennifer Radden is Professor Emerita in the Department of Philosophy at the University of Massachusetts, Boston. Radden's research is focused on philosophical issues arising out of mental health concepts and policy, and psychiatric practice. She is past president of the Association for the Advancement of Philosophy and Psychiatry, and her published work includes *The Nature of Melancholy: From Aristotle to Kristeva*. She edited *The Philosophy of Psychiatry: A Companion* (2004).

Nuria Sánchez Madrid is Associate Professor at the Faculty of Philosophy of the University Complutense of Madrid, Spain. She is a member of the CFUL (Lisbon) and of the IREPH of the University of Paris-Ouest, France. Her previous publications include "A civilização como destino: Kant e as formas da civilização" (2016) and an edited volume with Larry Krasnoff and Paula Satne, *Kant's Doctrine of Right in the Twenty First Century* (forthcoming).

Carlos Siopa is a PhD student and clinical researcher at the at the Lisbon Medical School, where he conducts work under the supervision of professor Telles Correia.

Diogo Telles Correia, MD, is a psychiatrist and invited teaching assistant at the Lisbon Medical School. He is the editor of *Acta Médica Portuguesa* and a fellow of the Portuguese Association for Behavioral and Cognitive Psychotherapy.

Introduction

Everyday and Non-everyday Delusions

Ana Falcato and Jorge Gonçalves

Human beings can be – and often are – deluded about the external world. What makes them come to be, remain, and in certain cases even *want to be* in such a state? And what does it ultimately mean to be deluded about the way the world is?

Whereas the idea of 'being deluded' about something or someone fits into common discourse, often used casually or unreflectively in daily life and linguistic exchanges, the very notion of 'delusion' is problematic from both a clinical and a philosophical standpoint.

When critically assessing the notion of delusion with an eye to both its current, daily uses and its significance in psychopathological contexts, it is helpful to begin by noting the extent to which a cluster of related but non-identical terms can have strikingly different meanings and trigger different mental associations.

Thus, to highlight the way in which even scientific terminology can foster ambiguities (especially regarding translation and local adaptation to clinical contexts) while nonetheless helping to refine meanings and clarify diagnostics, let us consider the key reference manual for the diagnosis and clinical assessment of mental disorders, the *Diagnostic and Statistical Manual of Mental Disorders* (DSM), published by the American Psychiatric Association.

In its fifth edition, published in 2013, delusions are classified as 'fixed beliefs that are not amenable to change in light of conflicting evidence'[1] and as '*thought-disruptions*, not necessarily akin to hallucinations'.[2]

It is noteworthy that scientists tend to define the mental phenomena at stake in privative or negative terms, but this meta-theoretical observation only shows how difficult it is to categorize these slippery events (or sets of mental events), which can both disturb and lend cohesion to our perceptive experiences and behavior. What this means, in turn, is that to the extent that perceptual delusions – akin to minor misperceptions – display to the perceiving eye something that isn't there to be seen, they can either help the

DOI: 10.4324/9781003288992-1

epistemic agent to compose or complete a visual scenario and make an inference about the world or lead to confusion and false assumptions about the external world.

When one turns from willed (or self-inflicted) forms of thought-disruption to non-willed or involuntary ones, the terminological and epistemic terrain changes as well. According to the DSM, 'delusion' must be distinguished from 'delirium' and 'hallucination' – the latter two being categorized as different 'neurocognitive disorders' that are equally unresponsive to external stimuli and which can reveal the onset of a serious and long-lasting mental pathology. *Delusions* would thus seem to be minor misapprehensions or miscalculations regarding the external world, with possible benefits to the subject thus affected, whereas *delirium* is a possible threshold of madness.

Even if the medical community employs a more or less stable definition of 'delirium', however, not all forms of delirium are linked to clinical contexts. Indeed, the specialized medical literature often contains other interpretations of this kind of mental disorder, typically unassociated with the pragmatic goal of a cure. In the DSM-5,[3] for instance, 'delirium' is associated with neurocognitive disorders that may develop into different diseases, sometimes irreversibly impairing cognitive functioning.[4]

In this book, we approach both delusions and an interrelated set of notions and mental phenomena with a wide range of analytical tools and from various theoretical standpoints. Among the many other strengths of the chapters collected in this volume is a conscious attempt to interpret delusions and delusional experiences within a *historical* framework.

The first part of the book – 'Historical Views, Contemporary Challenges' – is designed to provide readers with an informed historical perspective on delusions, including their individual and societal impact on mental health and power structures across cultures, while carefully examining the contemporary relevance of a set of historic accounts of delusion.

In Chapter 1, 'The Conceptual History of *Délire* (Delusion) from Its Appearance to the Present Day', Diogo Telles Correia and Carlos Siopa offer a synopsis of the meaning and use of the notion of 'delirium' in the history of modern medicine and psychopathology. Originating from the Latin word *delirare* ('out of normality' or 'away from the thread'), 'delirium' has never been uniformly understood by the European medical community. Through an examination of the evolution of a cluster of concepts in different European languages, the authors show that the medical community has never agreed on the precise meaning of the different notions used to account for mental diseases. They also show that the relatively recent agreement regarding the meaning of 'delusion' has not been unanimous in the history of medicine and may be no more than a useful scholarly device for dealing with heterogeneous phenomena.

Núria Sanchez Madrid's 'Kant on Mental Disorder and Pragmatic Delusions: Social Intercourse as Inhibitor of Lunacy' (Chapter 2) focuses on Kant's approach to delusion, developed in several texts under such headings as *Schein, Illusion* and *Täuschung*. Sanchez Madrid's chapter provides an account of Kant's treatment of the power that illusion holds over the human mind and the social world, arguing that Kant's approach shifts over time from the analysis of delusory operations within the 'battlefield' of metaphysics to the realm of anthropological interaction. While Kant understands the human capacity to be deluded as one of the drives that led to the establishment of social order, he consistently regards mental disorder as a pathology that should be eliminated from society, ideally with the help of social intercourse and its potential to relieve mental disorder. The chapter's principal conclusion is that Kant addresses metaphysical illusion as a symptom of the civilizing and moral function that this phenomenon fulfils in society. While reality appears as the central source of orientation, it is illusion that allows the subject to tolerate this reality without slipping into bewilderment and depression.

In Chapter 3 – 'The Madness of Guilt: Against Contemporary Approaches to Shame and Guilt' – Ana Falcato proposes a renewed approach to a half-forgotten text in contemporary studies on moral emotions, broadly understood: Eric Dodds's *The Greeks and the Irrational.* Overlooked in present-day and twentieth-century philosophical discussions of the relevance of emotions in moral deliberation, Dodds's book contains a remarkable (if half-hidden within philological material) model to account for what is wrong with guilt, in both classical and contemporary worldviews. Based on an insightful analysis of the cultural shift from *shame-cultures* to *guilt-cultures*, the central aim of this essay is to highlight the damaging effects of guilt on one's moral outlook and one's ethical actions.

Jennifer Radden's 'Ancient, Medieval and Early Modern Ideas about Delusional Thought in Burton's *Anatomy*' (Chapter 4), discusses Robert Burton's *Anatomy of Melancholy* in relation to contemporary models that aim to account for melancholy, or those delusions that are produced by the overlapping of different mental faculties, such as the imagination and reason. Radden's chapter provides an impressive historical account of the context in which Burton wrote the *Anatomy* and the set of conclusions he drew from observed features of the mentally infirmed, which he presents as social vignettes of seventeenth-century Britain. In the second half of the essay, Radden compares Burton's conclusions with contemporary models for interpreting delusional states in the philosophy of mind and within the brain sciences.

In the second part of the book – 'Varieties of Everyday Delusion' – the authors present and elaborate on contemporary views of delusions and their impact on mental life in general and on emotional balance more specifically. This is clearly connected to the first section of the book, and useful theoretical bridges are built between new and empirically informed views of delusions and their historical backgrounds and inspirations.

'Meaning and Delusion', by Rick Bellaar and Jasper Feyaerts (Chapter 5) is a thorough attempt to analyse delusions in a Wittgensteinian key. The authors build a careful argument in favor of a non-doxastic approach to delusions, claiming that the kind of irrationality that marks primary delusions consists in secondary sensical language, which presupposes forms of Wittgensteinian objective certainties, that is, those kinds of norms that are *constitutive* of knowledge. Thus, and going for a linguistic approach to the phenomena under analysis, Bellaar and Feyaerts claim that delusional language can be thought to consist of meaningful *avowals* of knowledge, rather than false, unwarranted or unverified beliefs.

In 'Delusional Realities, World Traveling and Transitional Objects' (Chapter 6), Shaun Gallagher and Ashleigh Morales approach delusions with a rich phenomenological toolkit. Building on the phenomenology of Alfred Schutz – and on William James's concept of 'sub-universes' – Gallagher and Morales conceive of delusional realities and experiences as detachments (often *useful* detachments) from the so-called paramount reality of the deluded subject. An interpretive model that makes sense of the many 'sub-universes' (cf. James) in which we live may be more useful for analyzing specifically deviant, pathological – and thus *delusional* – experiences than a strictly epistemological account that reduces delusions to false beliefs. Drawing on such phenomenological and psychiatric notions as 'world-travelling' and 'transitional objects', Morales and Gallagher situate the delusional experience on a continuum with other 'parallel realities' that make up our common social life.

In Chapter 7 – 'Minimal Biological Adaptiveness and the Phenomenology of Delusions in Schizophrenia' – Pablo López-Silva argues that delusions play a minimally adaptive role in schizophrenia, from a biological standpoint. Noting that beliefs are said to be *psychologically* adaptive when their adoption helps a subject to deal with psychologically problematic stimuli but are said to be *biologically* adaptive when their adoption increases one's chances of survival in a specific environment, López-Silva considers the subtle empirical conditions in which delusions are held in schizophrenia and argues that they play a key role within the survival mechanisms adopted by patients.

In Chapter 8, 'An Active Inference Account of the Cotard Delusion of Inexistence', Philip Gerrans makes a case for the importance of a neurocognitive approach to delusions. This chapter uses the Cotard delusion as a case study of an approach to the mind inspired by an 'active inference' approach to cognition. Gerrans argues that such an approach must start from a comprehensive description of the cognitive processes underlying the clinical phenomenology of delusion-formation and delusional behavior and, from that point, trace the genesis of delusions from neurobiology to phenomenology and back.

Finally, in the third part of the book – 'The Normative Framework of Delusion' – the authors explore normative frameworks for categorizing delusions and analyze the impact of delusions on the daily lives of subjects and their caregivers.

Filipe Arantes-Gonçalves and Georg Northoff's 'From Abnormal Time-Space Experience to Delusions – Spatiotemporal Psychopathology' (Chapter 9) offers a phenomenological account of the primary role of space and time in the development of delusional experiences, particularly in patients with schizophrenia. The authors argue that delusions, as well as hallucinations, develop as symptomatic consequences of a set of distorted experiences of the outside world in which patients project internally oriented thought contents onto the external world.

In Chapter 10 – 'Defining Delusion in the DSM-5' – Jorge Gonçalves defends a philosophical reading of the *Diagnostic and Statistical Manual of Mental Disorders* (the DSM-5), a central text in the fields of psychiatry and neuroscience. Gonçalves criticizes strict clinical readings of the definition of 'delusion' in the DSM-5 for their lack of nuance, instead advocating a mixed interpretation of delusions as both beliefs *and* experiences.

In 'Delusions across and beyond Diagnoses' (Chapter 11), Lisa Bortolotti and Luigi Grassi examine the heterogeneity that marks the origin, development and behavioral consequences of delusions. The authors firmly stress the unviability of isolating the unifying and defining features of delusions (as a set of necessary and sufficient conditions), given the heterogeneity of manifestations of delusional thought and behavior across the clinical and non-clinical population. Bortolotti and Grassi argue that it is important, from a theoretical standpoint, to insist on the overwhelming relevance of the *incorrigibility* of delusional thought in the face of contrary evidence rather than arguing for a systematic definition of delusions as false beliefs or belief systems.

The wide-ranging theoretical landscape on the nature and function of delusions is evidence of the richness of the phenomena under examination, as well as the fruitfulness of continuously updating the models we rely on to account for delusional experiences – in both the medical and the non-medical community.

This book will be of interest to scholars from a broad range of disciplines – including historians, psychiatrists, philosophers, psychologists, healthcare workers and caregivers – insofar as it brings together readings of delusions and related mental and moral phenomena as they have developed in the history of ideas, putting them in conversation with an informed, original discussion of the impact of everyday delusions on agents' moral lives and the *Lebenswelt* they inhabit or come to inhabit – often due to so-called delusional states.

Notes

1 American Psychiatric Association. *Diagnostic and Statistical Manual of Mental Disorders*, 5th Edition. Washington, DC: American Psychiatric Association, 2013 (p. 87).
2 Idem, p. 819.
3 Cf. DSM-5 (2013).
4 See DSM-5, 2013: 591: 'The neurocognitive disorders (NCDs) (referred to in DSM-IV as "Dementia, Delirium, Amnestic, and Other Cognitive Disorders") begin with delirium, followed by the syndromes of major NCD, mild NCD, and their etiological subtypes. The major or mild NCD subtypes are NCD due to Alzheimer's disease; vascular NCD; NCD with Lewy bodies; NCD due to Parkinson's disease; frontotemporal NCD; NCD due to traumatic brain injury; NCD due to HIV infection; substance/medication-induced NCD; NCD due to Huntington's disease; NCD due to prion disease; NCD due to another medical condition; NCD due to multiple etiologies; and unspecified NCD. The NCD category encompasses the group of disorders in which the primary clinical deficit is in cognitive function, and that are acquired rather than developmental. Although cognitive deficits are present in many if not all mental disorders (e.g., schizophrenia, bipolar disorders), only disorders whose core features are cognitive are included in the NCD category. The NCDs are those in which impaired cognition has not been present since birth or very early life, and thus represents a decline from a previously attained level of functioning'.

References

American Psychiatric Association. *Diagnostic and Statistical Manual of Mental Disorders*, 5th Edition. Washington, DC: American Psychiatric Association, 2013.

Bortolotti, Lisa (Ed.) *Delusions in Context*. London: Palgrave Macmillan, 2018.

Williams, Bernard. *Problems of the Self: Philosophical Papers 1956–1972*. Cambridge: Cambridge University Press, 1973.

Part I

Historical Views, Contemporary Challenges

1 The Conceptual History of *Délire* (Delusion) from Its Appearance to the Present Day

Diogo Telles Correia and Carlos Siopa

Introduction

The importance of *délire* is central in psychopathology, with Jaspers going so far as to state "*délire* was at all times the fundamental phenomenon of madness". Etymologically the term *délire* derives from the Latin word *delirare* (de – outside; lirare, lira – plow furrow). This is the origin of the term used by Latin countries (France, Italy, Spain, Portugal), referring to individuals who deviate from normality.[1] These facts explain why *délire* has taken on several meanings other than thought disorders over history.

The term *delusion*, used in English-speaking countries, has a different origin (from the Latin *delude* – belief/ false opinion), referring since the 15th century to a falsification of the content of thought. In the *Royal Chronicle of Fabyan* (1494), there is a reference to this term as "an act of deceiving".[2] At the Congress of Paris in 1950, there were attempts to universalize the term *delusion*, suppressing the other synonyms in the different languages, but to no avail.[3]

The German term *Wahn* emerges in the 18th century, meaning uncertain assumptions and insecurity regarding what might happen. This later came to acquire the meaning of unreal belief and judgment confusion, as opposed to rational judgment.[2]

Hence, while the terms *delusion* and *Wahn* have, in their origin, a denotation of content of thought disorder, in the sense of an unrealistic belief, the term *délire* derives from the designation of something that departs from normality, from the expected, not initially referring to thought disorder. This relates to the dispersed evolution of this concept throughout the history of psychiatry, as will be later addressed.

The term *delirium* was used as a synonym of *délire* until the late-19th century, having later been renamed as acute confusional syndrome, mainly due to Anglo-Saxon influence.

Parallel to other psychopathological concepts, *délire* had a complex evolution before reaching the restricted meaning it is known for nowadays.

DOI: 10.4324/9781003288992-3

Originally, it had a broader meaning (when *délire* and mental illness were synonymous), but nowadays it refers to a mere thought disorder in the psychopathological examination. Henceforth, studying the diachrony of *délire* is fundamental for the global understanding of psychopathology history. In this chapter, we explore the conceptual history of *délire* in psychopathology, from the dawn of time up to modernity.

Before the 18th century

The history of delirium and madness are inevitably linked. After the Middle Ages and at the beginning of the Age of Enlightenment, the deistic notion was gradually replaced by a more rational and scientific approach. Mad people were no longer thought to be possessed by malignant spirits and began to be seen as sick. Thomas Hobbes (1588–1679), an English philosopher, stated "the opinions about madness that were formulated in ancient and modern times are two. Some say it derives from passion, and others, that it proceeds from demons and spirits". He defended the first, stating "all passions that produce a strange behavior different from ordinary are given the general name of madness". Nevertheless, he believed madness was not always accompanied by agitation or behavioral exaltation "if a man in an asylum threatens us with their discreet conversation, and as we said goodbye we asked him who he was and he told us that he was God the Father, we would not need to observe any extravagant behavior to confirm his madness", thus being the badge of madness we would designate today as thought content disorder (*délire*).[2] However, it was Pedro de Heredia (1579–1655), a Spanish doctor at the court of Felipe IV, who writes a medical treatise on "*délire*", published posthumously by his disciple, Pedro de Astorga. Here, the author emphasizes the importance of reason: "when a man follows his intellect, he acts rationally, if not the case, he strands from reason. This reason is the main power that rules and governs all others, and whose maladjusted activity is *délire*."[2] According to this author, reasoning could suffer an imbalance that manifests itself psychopathologically through *délire*. He goes further concerning the characterization of *délire*: "*délire*, in general, follows the direction of an imbalance, but the way of *délire* depends on the patient's previous personality". In this way, the author foresaw much of what would come to develop on this topic.

The *Encyclopédie*, in 1754, defines *délire* as an "error of judgment during wakefulness". It applies the word *delirium* as a synonym for *délire* and further characterizes it concerning the presence or absence of fever, assuming its causes to be organic: "the soul is always in the same state and is not susceptible to change. So, the present error of judgment in *délire* cannot be attributed to the soul but rather to the disposition of bodily organs".[4]

The importance of *délire* to the definition of madness was a constant among 18th-century authors. However, its distinction from other psychopathological phenomena (according to current canons), such as hallucinations, remained difficult. William Battie (1703–1776), an English physician, defines madness based on *délire*, reiterating the importance of this psychopathological disorder closely associated with hallucinations:

> No one doubts that the perception of objects that do not really exist or that do not correspond really to the senses can be a sure sign of madness. Therefore, the imagination from *délire* is not only something indisputable but the essential character of madness. … [H]e who is properly mad is totally and unalterably persuaded of the existence or appearance of something unreal or that is not before him, but he still behaves according to such an erroneous persuasion.[5]

For Vicenzo Chiarugi (1759–1820), an Italian physician, *délire* was the paradigm of madness, as he further examined it:

> in the first place an erroneous judgment consists of establishing a relationship between things in disagreement to the correct opinion expressed by man's common sense. Second, some false perceptions arise, without necessarily existing a sensory defect. Finally, in the mind of people with *délire*, certain sudden and extravagant associations occur.[6]

Nevertheless, at this point, some authors were already concerned with differentiating thought disorder (*délire*) and perception disorder (hallucinations) (as understood today). Thomas Arnold (1742–1816), of the Leicester Asylum in London, wrote a prodigious work (*Observations on the Nature, Kinds, Causes and Prevention of Insanity*), where he intended to describe and classify symptoms of madness. He differentiated *Ideal insanity* from *Notional insanity*. While the first was defined as a "state in which a person imagines he sees, hears, perceives or talks to people or things that don't have an external existence for his senses at that moment", the second corresponds to the

> mental state in which a person sees, hears or perceive external objects as they exist but has notions of powers, properties … of things, people, of himself and others, who seem rude, erroneous and unreasonable for the common sense of the sober and sane part of mankind".[7]

This author shows discontent with the struggle to define *délire/delirium*: "the term *delirium* has been universally adopted. … However, it has been given different definitions according to the various authors, having many not defined it at all, and none as well as would be desirable".[7] He underlines an Anglo-Saxon trend to find a restrictive term for that concept, which was later achieved by abandoning the term *délire* when describing thought disorder, having then opted for *delusion*.

Alexander Crichton (1763–1856), who also practiced medicine in England, divided the diseased notions into two groups:

> Firstly there are diseased perceptions attributed by the patient to some object from external senses, as when he believes he sees, hears, tastes or smells things that have no real existence. ... [S]econdly there are abstract notions referring to people's qualities, conditions, things and to their relationship with them, like when he imagines his friends conspired to kill him, or that he is condemned to beg.

This author also broke with John Locke's notion (among others) that misperceptions invariably led to *délire* (as we understand them today).[3]

According to Johan Heinroth (1773–1843), a German physician, *délire* (*Wahn*), was the "madness core and basic disorder (*Verrucktheit*)", although this author considered troubles of the soul to cause madness.[8] He belonged to the "psychologistics" trend, whom Germán Elías Berrios prefers to call the "psychics", which dominated German psychiatry at the end of the 18th century/beginning of the 19th, according to which mental illness reflected the state of the incorporeal soul. Most of these authors related madness to ethical-religious factors. According to Pierre Pichot, this trend might have delayed German psychiatry evolution at that time, as compared to other countries. It would later be opposed by the "somatics", a fundamental trend in establishing psychiatry as a science, of which stands out Wilhelm Griesinger, who stated that mental illness is a brain disease.[9]

After the 18th Century

After the 18th century, definitions of the concept *délire* were further diversified, and therefore different positions were established among French, German and English authors. These two last groups adopted once and for all the more restrictive terms to describe thought content disorder, which corresponds to what we recognize today as *délire* (*Wahn* for the Germans and *delusion* for the English).

France

At the end of the 18th century, the term *délire* related to different aspects like madness in general (which included disorders of thought, perception, emotions and affects, psychomotricity, among others) or *délire per se* (as we understand it today, as a disorder of thought). The terms *délire* and *delirium* were used as synonyms, and the *délire* that resulted from madness only differed from the organic variant by the absence of fever.

Philippe Pinel, an author from the turn of the 18th century to the 19th century, divided mental illnesses in a monolithic manner with few mental symptoms' specifications. In his *Medical-Philosophical Treatise about mental alienation or mania*, he established four categories: mania, melancholy, dementia and idiotism. Mania was distinguished from melancholy since the last refers to a partial form of madness, restricted only to some areas and only with repercussions in some aspects of life. It characterizes a type of manic state as "*folie raisonante*", or mania without *délire*, with conservation of intellectual faculties and only emotional disorders remaining. Regarding mania without *délire*, he notes that "the person ... enjoys his free exercise of reason, even during his attacks, responding directly to asked questions and not having any inconsistency of ideas, no sign of *délire*". Here we find the definition of *délire* closely related to a reasoning disorder, despite his writings often assuming *délire* as synonymous with madness in general.[10]

Augustin Landré-Beauvais (1772–1840), a medical semiology specialist, writes in 1813 the book *Séméiotique ou traité des signes des maladies*, in which he describes *délire* in the section of *signs related to understanding ability*: "The deviance of human understanding functions leads, in the first place, to the patient's association between incompatible ideas and to taking as truth their combinations; these constitute different forms of *délire*. In the second place, the patient develops false ideas relating to one or more types of objects." The author also classified brain disease–associated *délire* as symptomatic *délire*.[2]

Jean-Étienne Esquirol (1772–1840) replaces the term "alienation" by "mental illness", in his 1838 work *Des maladies mentales considerés sous rapports medical, hygienique et medico-legal*. He officiated the concept of madness as a type of disease and designated monomania as a set of partial madness conditions (which would then replace Pinel's melancholy), as opposed to the term *mania* ("a type of more generalized madness").[11]

According to this author, the difference between *délire* and hallucination is not clear. In the *Packouke* dictionary (1814) he writes the following: "A man develops *délire* when his feelings are not connected to external objects, when his ideas are not connected to his feelings, when his judgments and decisions are independent of his will". Alexandre Bottex skillfully describes that, for Esquirol, the term *hallucination* meant "a *délire* in which individuals believe they are having senses without there being an external object".[12]

Jean-Pierre Falret (1794–1870) kept a comprehensive notion of *délire*: "*délire* includes, in general, all disorders of intelligence whatever the cause, origin and duration; therefore, it cannot be used to name a symptom (common to many diseases) or some well-defined disease". As traditional among French authors of his time, he does not distinguish between *délire* and hallucination: "The numerous connections that hallucinations present regarding other *délire* symptoms are many"; "current science tends to look at these phenomena (hallucinations) as intelligence disorders".[13] This author also mentions that "the main feature of *délire* corresponds to its lack of morbid character awareness from which the patient suffers and which he can never recognize without halting of *délire*".[13]

This multidimensional vision of *délire* would come to be followed by many French authors throughout the 19th century, unlike the more intellectualist Anglo-Saxon vision of *délire*. This stance is wisely exposed by Étienne-Jean Georget (1795–1828), a disciple of Pinel and Esquirol, who claims that: "the available definitions of *délire* are vague, unintelligible".[2]

Joseph Guislain (1797–1860) introduces a clearer definition of *délire*: "aberration of reason, chronic error of concepts and a disorder of ideas against which the patient cannot fight; understanding as real what is only just phantoms of his imagination." The author classified *délire* as being general (if compromising all ideas) or special (affecting only a few: mono*délire*). He also proposed one of the earliest classifications of *délire* regarding its content (persecutory, inspirational [erotic, religious, ambitious, hypochondriac], metamorphic [believing to be something one's not] and hallucinatory). He also does not distinguish *délire* from hallucination.[14]

Jules Baillarger (1809–1890) was the first author to describe a concept close to what we now call delusional perceptions. He states that the difference between false judgments secondary to normal sensations and secondary to illusions is that in the first case there was no illusion since the perception was normal. Hence, here the patients "interpret in a particular way" a reality-based sensation, making false judgments and developing "a delusional idea out of a normal sensation".[15]

Jacques-Joseph Moreau de Tours (1804–1884), based on his observations of people intoxicated with psychoactive drugs who developed hallucinations and *délire*, establishes a theory of a *continuum* between normality and alienation.[16]

At the end of the 19th century, a successive professionalization of French alienism took place with the institution *Societé Medico–Psychologique*, the publication of the *Annales medico-psychologiques* (1843, first issue) and with thematic discussion sessions.[4] Jules Cotard (1840–1889) presents his works in these sessions, regarding *délire des negations*, a set of several symptoms: (1) delusional ideas of the non-existence of all or parts of the person; (2) depressed mood with severe anxiety symptoms; (3) suicidal ideation; (4) damnation or possession ideas; (5) pain insensitivity; (6) immortality ideas (Telles-Correia, 2013). This *délire* constitutes a multidimensional syndrome, as was usual to the French approach of the time.

Charles Lasègue (1816– 1883) describes the term "persecutory delusion" (*délire of persecutions*), which he later names chronic *délire*. He divides it into four periods: incubation, organization and dementia or terminal phase.[17]

Certain authors such as Paul Garnier (1848–1905) mention that persecutory *délire* becomes grandiose *délire*. Others oppose Laségue's theory regarding progression to dementia.[2]

Garnier proposes a latent period in which the first subtle manifestations of *délire* take place. This period composes a pre-delusional state precursor as we understand it today.

Auguste Axenfeld (1825–1876) divided *délire* into two classes: (1) *délire de paroles* (characterized by incoherent verborreic speech) and (2) *délire de action* (ambulatory madness – *folie ambulatoire*, characterized by disorganized behavior, as we understand it today).[2]

Benjamin Ball (1822–1893) and Antoine Ritti (1844–1920) unveiled a widely general definition of *délire*: "every psychic morbid disorder that affect[s] the intellectual, sentimental, actions and will scopes" (*délire sensoriel, délire de la penseé, délire de sentiments, délire des acts*).[1]

Jules Séglas (1856–1939) emphasized that one of the main features of *délire* is that the patient "holds these ideas as true, without prior certification and with an absolute lack of insight". He divides every *délire* into three groups, based on its psychopathological characteristics: *délire* of inference or interpretation (the patient formulates a *délire* based on his reasoning, passing through all the logical phases of thought but with false premises and erroneous conclusions), *délire* of immediate perception (which originate from illusions and hallucinations), *délire* of verbal symbols (based on formal associative links). On the other hand, this author also classifies *délire* based on its content, distinguishing several themes such as self-accusation, persecution, grandiosity, hypochondria, negation and the like.[18]

Phillippe Chaslin (1857–1923) published in 1912 his work *Elements de sémiologie et clinique mentales*, describing concepts such as hallucination, delusional perception (defined initially by Baillarger and later developed by Karl Jaspers, Kurt Shneider and Hans Gruhle), obsession and so forth. For him, *délire* and hallucination had the same psychological and neurophysiological origin and often appeared together. He mentions that *délire* can occur as isolated and disconnected (in *dementia praecox*, for example) or create a system of ideas (for example, in *paranoia*).

Germany

Authors such as Ernst von Feuchtersleben (1806–1849) define *délire* (*Wahn*) as something more restricted. *Wahn* supposes "the erroneous combination of a set of ideas, often united with the patient's own inclinations, without being aware of the error or even able to overcome it. These ideas yield insane actions and speeches". Wilhelm Griesinger (1817–1868) agreed with von Feuchtersleben when describing delusional ideas (*Wahnideen*) as false contents of thought. He considered them as "symptoms", distinguishing them from other erroneous beliefs.[2] The first copy of the *Archiv für Psychiatrie und Nervenkrankheiten* was edited in 1867, by its founder Wilhem Griesenger, who criticized contemporary German psychiatry as he considered it alienated from philosophical and religious questions, highlighting that psychiatric disorders are parallel to neurological and medical diseases and considered histopathological research as fundamental. His precept "psychiatric disorders are brain disorders", accurately translates his outlook. This would become the perspective of several Germans at the end of the 19th century, such as Franz Nissl and Alois Alzheimer. Thus, descriptive psychopathology was only further developed in the early 20th century, after Jaspers.

Jaspers (1883–1969) published his *General Psychopathology* in 1913, where he develops the phenomenological method. For Jaspers, phenomenology attends to intuitively access the subjective psychic states that patients experience, delineate them, distinguish them as strictly as possible and apply them in precise manners.[19] On these grounds, he classifies most sharply the many groups of psychopathological phenomena. "According to Jaspers, it was impossible to order and classify phenomenological findings in a systematically satisfactory manner at that time. ... But in some way, it was essential to order them provisionally".[19] For Jaspers, the best organization was based on the deepest disparities among the phenomena. He suggested these groups: object awareness (perception disorders), space-time experience, body awareness, reality awareness (*délire* and delusional ideas), affective states, impulse and will, self-awareness and reflective phenomena. Many groups endured until modern times, keeping or changing their names, while others were suppressed. He describes each concept grouped in those sections, including delusional ideas.[19] Berrios draws attention to the fact that many of his definitions are based on what was developed by his contemporary and predecessor psychopathologists, mostly of the French school.[2] He classifies delusional ideas as false judgments, characterized by (1) irreducible before logic, argumentation or collective opinion; (2) plain conviction (subjective certainty independent of experience); (3) impossible content. He also distinguishes between true delusional ideas (*echte Wahnideen*) – being primary delusional ideas – from deliroid ideas (*wahnafte ideen*), including overvalued ideas and secondary delusions. In the group of primary delusional experiences, he characterizes delusional perception, delusional representation (corresponding to Kurt Schneider's delusional memory) and delusional cognition (a term K. Schneider considered as ambiguous).[19, 20] Gruhle (1880–1958) further develops several forms of primary delusion which he defines as delusional mood, delusional perception (according to Jaspers) and delusional occurrence. K. Schneider (1887–1967) divides the concept of primary delusion into delusional perception, delusional occurrence and delusional memory (of a delusional perception type or a delusional occurrence type).[20]

Emil Kraepelin (1856–1926), particularly interested in nosology, divided psychoses into *dementia praecox*, manic-depressive psychosis and *paranoia*. This last one is a "delusion of insidious beginning and chronic evolution deriving from internal causes ... and without personality deterioration".[4] Ernst Kretschmer develops the term *paranoia*, in which he considers the *délire* to be produced "by the cumulative actions of typical vital experiences or situations on characterological and constitutional bases", underlining its psychological comprehensibility.[2]

England

English Psychiatry was heavily influenced by the French school until the 19th century. However, since the 18th century, authors like Arnold opposed the use of the term *délire/delirium* to describe a symptom.

Echoing this stance, William Tuke (1827–1895) composed a manual and dictionary at the end of the 19th century regarding medical psychology, where he describes *délire* as a "term used by the French to describe *delirium* as well as mania and monomania", expressing the conceptual scope associated to the term *délire* as considered by the French school of this time.[21] Concerning the term *delirium*, he describes it as a syndrome associated with *délire* and hallucinations (in today's sense of the terms) and secondary to an underlying medical illness. The term *delusion* is used synonymously with *insane ideas*, being separated from hallucinations in the psychopathological examination. This Anglo-Saxon point of view was the most popular in psychiatric literature until today.

Discussion and Conclusion

Etymologically, the term "delusion" is based on the Latin word *delirare* (de – outside; lirare, lira – plow furrow), referring to individuals who depart from normality. This explains the fact why the term *délire* has, throughout history, acquired several meanings other than thought disorders.

Before the 18th century, several authors drew attention to the importance of the content of thought disorders and reason disorders (in the way we understand delusions today), for the definition of madness.

There have been several attempts to define *délire* in the history of modern medicine and psychopathology. Pedro de Heredia (1579–1655) for example, states that "reason is the main power that rules and governs all others, and whose maladjusted activity is *délire*". Since the beginning of medical classification, *délire* was synonymous with madness in general, and not a symptom, as it later came to be. In the 19th century, there was still some confusion among French authors, the most influencing psychiatric trend at that time, who interpreted *délire* as a syndrome that involved several psychopathological changes beyond thought disorders, particularly persisting the closeness between thought disorders and perception disorders (hallucinations). The terms *délire* and *delirium* were used as a synonym, and the *délire* of madness only differed from organic *délire* by the absence of fever.

These terms have different origins and paths – the English term *delusion* and the German term *Wahn*, which came to replace the terms *délire* and *delirium* for a more restricted designation of content of thought disorders, bearing proof of such historical nuances. The new terminology in a way expressed the discontentment of the English and Germans with the vagueness of the French concept of *délire*, in the 18th century.

On the other hand, the development of the concept of *délire*, as we understand it today, had several contributions long before the one that's considered the most important, the one from Jaspers who characterized it and classified it masterfully.

Joseph Guislan (1797–1860) defined delusional ideas by underlining their characteristic unshakable conviction; Falret (1794–1870) underlines the lack of insight in these patients; Baillarger (1809–1890) came near the concept of delusional perception for the first time (which would later be developed by Chaslin, Jaspers and K. Schneider); Lasègue (1816–1883) spoke of dementia for the first time, after the evolution of chronic *délire*; Garnier (1848–1905) describes latency periods before the development of the *délire* itself (approaching pre-delusional states that would come to develop in the future); Séglas (1856–1939) underlines that one of the main characteristics of *délire* is that the patient "holds these ideas as true, without prior certification and with an absolute lack of insight" and based on its content he distinguishes several themes. Chaslin (1857–1923) specifies simple and systematic types of *délire*.

In Germany, from the turn of the 19th century to the 20th century, Jaspers (1883–1969) characterized and classified *délire*, according to what is currently settled, heavily based on his predecessor francophone authors.

Later, Gruhle (1880–1958) and Kurt Schneider (1887–1967) provided developments on the definition of types of primary delusions.

In England, at end of the 19th century, Tuke (1827–1895) composed a manual and dictionary of medical psychology, where he describes *délire* as a "term used by the French to describe *delirium* as well as mania and monomania" – in this way expressing the difficulty that the French had in defining this term (already announced by Arnold in the 18th century). Concerning the term *delirium*, he describes it as a syndrome associated with *délire* and hallucinations (in today's sense of the terms) and secondary to an underlying medical illness. The term *delusion* is used synonymously with *insane ideas*, being separated from hallucinations in the psychopathological examination. The term *delusion* was never internationalized, even though that had been tried in the Congress of Paris in 1950. This Anglo-Saxon point of view was the most popular in psychiatric literature until today.

This review approached the most relevant authors and highlighted the difficult delineation between the concepts of *délire* and thought disorders and all other psychopathological disorders, namely perception disorders (hallucinations), which remain in conceptual juxtaposition until the end of the 19th century.

It is essential to develop studies on the evolution of psychopathology concepts, to a sharper and deeper reflection on current psychopathological semiology.

Conflicting Interests

The author declares no conflict of interest.

Funding

The author received no financial support for the research, authorship, and/or publication of this article.

References

1. Berrios, Germán e Fuentenebro Filiberto, Delirios. In Rogelio Luque e Villagrán, José. *Psicopatología Descriptiva: Nuevas Tendencias*. Madrid: Trotta; 2000. p. 337–358.
2. Berrios, Gérman e Fuentenebro Filiberto, Historia Conceptual del Delirio Antes del Siglo XIX. In Gérman Berrios e Fuentenebro Filiberto ed. *Delirio, Historia, Clinica Metateoría*. Madrid: Trotta; 1996. p. 23–95.
3. Berrios, Germán, Delusions. In Berrios, Germán ed. *The History of Mental Symptoms*. Cambridge: Cambridge University Press; 1996. p. 85–139.

4. Olivos, Patricio, La mente delirante. Psicopatologia del delírio. *Rev Chil Neuro-Psiquiat.* 2009; 47 (1), p. 67–85.
5. Battie, William, *A Treatise on Madness.* London: J. Whiston and B White; 1758.
6. Chiarugi, Vicenzo, *On Insanity and its Classification.* Trans by G. Mora Canton: Science History Publications; 1987.
7. Arnold, Thomas, *Observations on the Nature, Kinds, Causes, and Preventions of Insanity, Lunacy or Madness.* Vol. II. Leicester: G Ireland; 1782.
8. Heinroth, Johan, *Textbook of Disturbances of Mental Life.* Trans by J. Schmorak. Baltimore: John Hopkins University Press; 1975.
9. Pichot, Pierre e Barahona Fernandes, *Um Século de Psiquiatria. A Escola Alemã de Psiquiatria.* Lisboa: Roche SA; 1984. p. 40–56.
10. Pinel, Philippe, *Tratado Médico-Filosófico sobre Alienação Mental.* Trans by B. Barreiros, N. Melim, N. Proença Lisboa: Ed. Colibri; 2011.
11. Esquirol, E., *Des maladies mentales considérées sous les rapports médical, hygienique et médico-legal.* Paris: Bailliére; 1838.
12. Bottex, A., *Essai sur les hallucinations.* Lyon: L. Perrin; 1836.
13. Falret, Jean, Délire. In *Des maladies mentales et des asiles d'aliénés.* Paris: B. Baillière; 1864.
14. Guislain, J., *Leçons orales sur les Phrenopathies ou Traité théorique et pratique des maladies mentales.* Gand: Ed. Hebbelynck; 1852.
15. Baillarger, J., *Recherches sur les maladies mentales.* Paris: Ed. Masson; 1890.
16. Moreau de Tours, J., *Du hachisch et de l'aniénation mentale.* Paris: Ed Masson; 1859.
17. Laségue, C., Du Délire des Pérsecutions. In *Archives génerales de medicine.* Vol. 28; 129–150. Paris: Labé; Panckoucke; 1852.
18. Séglas, J., Séméiologie des affections mentales. In Ballet, G. ed. *Traité de Pathologie mentale.* Paris: Doin; 1903.
19. Jaspers, K., *General Psychopathology.* Trans by M. Hamilton, J. Hoening 7th German Edition. Manchester: Manchester University Press; 1963.
20. Telles-Correia, D., Guerreiro, D., Barbosa, A., Semiologia psicopatológica. In *Manual de Psicopatologia.* Lisboa: Lidel; 2013.
21. Tuke, Daniel, *A Dictionary of Psychological Medicine.* Philadelphia: P. Blakiston, Son & Co.; 1892

2 Kant on Mental Disorder and Pragmatic Delusions

Social Intercourse as Inhibitor of Lunacy

Nuria Sánchez Madrid

Introduction

Kant devoted a standing attention throughout his writings to the phenomenon of *delusion*, a concept that is analysed in his writings through the use of terms such as *Schein*, *Illusion* and *Täuschung*. This chapter attempts to give an account of Kant's treatment of the power that illusion holds over the human mind and of the value it receives from the social world, arguing that Kant's approach moves from inspecting delusory operations within the "battlefield" of metaphysics to check out how they work in the realm of anthropological interaction. The chapter has the following structure. First, I tackle Kant's reading of illusion in the *Critique of Pure Reason*, as a common phenomenon throughout the history of philosophy, which no philosophical school has been able to unravel. Moreover, I address Kant's appeal to critique as a methodological tool that constitutes a mature reaction to delusion ensuing from the entanglement of the human mind in its repeated attempt to grasp unreachable objects. My aim in this section is to illustrate some of the consequences that result from Kant's association of illusion with the nature of reason, which also stakes the hope that strong mental discipline is able to mitigate the threat of illusion. Second, I break down the map of mental illnesses Kant displays in the second book of the *Anthropology from a Pragmatic Point of View* (1798), letting aside the phenomenon of hypochondria, which the author dissects independently from psychological derangement. In this section, I furthermore claim that Kant understands mental disorder as the belief to live in an illusory world after the subject has lost common sense, which keeps her mental activity tied to objective phenomena. Third, I consider the shift that Kant undertakes in his anthropological writings, in which he also examines the realm of illusion and delusion, yet this time as a constitutive and fertile part of the socialization process. In his *Anthropology*, Kant views delusion as a metaphor for the maturation the human nature has to achieve and investigates the moral role that civilizing deception fulfils within the social world.

DOI: 10.4324/9781003288992-4

Accordingly, in the third section, I examine Kant's interpretation of the alternating cycle of illusion and delusion as part of the process of becoming fully human, a process that forestalls falling prey to mental illness. While Kant understands the human capacity to be deluded as one of the drives making social order more resilient, he consistently regards *mental disorder* as a pathology that should be removed from society with the help of social intercourse and its potential to relieve mental disorder. Finally, I discuss why, while social illusion and delusion are seen as key factors for strengthening social normativity, mental illness is viewed as a threat to the social world. The principal conclusion I draw from this exploration is that illusion, according to Kant, fosters social intercourse and social enjoyment as a therapy for bewilderment and depression. Thus, one can say that Kant understands social intercourse as closely tied to illusory phenomena, even if the first brings the latter under control and uses them as tools to make life a more entertaining enterprise.

Borders of the Mind and Mental Disorder in Kant

As is well known, Kant chooses a geographical image to depict how reason must be able to guide itself amidst the greatest illusions and deceptions. According to this account, to determine the borders of legitimate knowledge for human understanding embodies a key task of the critical project.[1] Moreover, to explore the faculties of the mind requires one to accurately draw the borders of their use, as it prevents us from wrongly applying them for obtaining knowledge. Borders also fulfil a central role in Kant's legal and political philosophy, insofar as they guarantee national sovereignty and simultaneously allow us to sketch what cosmopolitan normativity should be, beyond the national sovereignty of the states. In a conclusive section of the *Prolegomena*, which furnishes a neat outline of the epistemic outcomes of the first *Critique*, Kant stresses a key distinction between *boundaries* (*Grenzen)* and *limits* (*Schranken*). For breaking down accurately what the human mind obtains through each one of the epistemic determinations, Kant argues for the enduring character of boundaries in contrast with the relative value of cognitive limits:

> *Boundaries* [*Grenzen*] (in extended things) always presuppose a space that is found outside a certain fixed location, and that encloses that location; *limits* [*Schranken*] require nothing of the kind, but are mere negations that affect a magnitude insofar as it does not possess absolute completeness.[2]

Notwithstanding that to lay down boundaries yields in a quite trustful way the scope of human faculties and cognition, this cognitive structure entails an extra space outside it, which is unable to be inspected by the understanding, thus bringing about logical seductions that misguide the epistemic progress. In this context, the Kantian subject might engage into a relation with boundaries that neglects the objective value of these logical milestones. As Kant highlights in the *Doctrine of Method* in the first *Critique*, there is a blatant distance between the fact of being convinced of the truth and objectivity of a claim and the fact of being merely persuaded of it, insofar as "*[p]ersuasion* is a mere semblance [*Schein*] since the ground of the judgment, which lies solely in the subject, is held to be objective" (KrV A 820/B 848). To put it differently, the human mind appears in this account as vulnerable enough to generate mistakes ensuing from illusions of the faculty of judgement, which confuses objective reasons with subjective impressions, giving birth to delusory approaches to the reality around.[3] Kant warns thus the readers of the first *Critique* to be wary in their cognitive procedures, so that the causes of epistemic mistake do not remain unnoticed to them. For preventing this sort of mistake, the attentive reader of transcendental philosophy is kindly recommended to apply all her attention to perform a sound cognitive synthesis, without taking subjective impressions for objective features of the real world. Naturally, with these pedagogical remarks Kant intends to foster the harmony among the faculties, without renouncing to warn against the dangers ensuing from the menacing "ocean of illusion" surrounding the land of truth. A well-known passage from the mentioned writing displays the state of doubt and anxiety piercing even the subject regardful to the rules and boundaries of an orderly understanding:

> We have now not only traveled through the land of pure understanding, and carefully inspected each part of it, but we have also surveyed it, and determined the place for each thing in it. But this land is an island, and enclosed in unalterable boundaries by nature itself. It is the land of truth (a charming name), surrounded by a broad and stormy ocean, the true seat of illusion, where many a fog bank and rapidly melting iceberg pretend to be new lands and, ceaselessly deceiving with empty hopes the voyager looking around for new discoveries, entwine him in adventures from which he can never escape and yet also never bring to an end.[4]

The evidence that the continent of truth is amidst an ocean of illusion does not widen the sort of objects that critical philosophy recognizes as possible epistemic targets. Quite on the contrary, the stock that the subject takes of the path she accomplished at the end of the *Transcendental Analytic* brings the outcome that "truth and illusion are not in the object, insofar as it is intuited, but in the judgment about it insofar as it is thought" (KrV A 293/B 350). In fact, as the senses do not judge in the epistemic process, the source of illusion must be assigned to another cause, as it is the case of "the relation of the object to our understanding" (ibid.). Thus, the seat of illusion does not draw to a concrete field of phenomena, but rather to an epistemic attitude oblivious to control the mistakes leading to false statements and conclusions. Yet Kant does not expect that a sheer discipline might remove the effects of "transcendental illusion", since it belongs to the very gist of reason and even seems to stem from the bottomless depths of this faculty, which thus easily passes subjective principles through objective ones:

> The transcendental dialectic will therefore content itself with uncovering the illusion in transcendental judgments, while at the same time protecting us from being deceived by it; but it can never bring it about that transcendental illusion (like logical illusion) should even disappear and cease to be an illusion. For what we have to do with here is a *natural* and unavoidable *illusion* which itself rests on subjective principles and passes them off as objective, whereas logical dialectic in its dissolution of fallacious inferences has to do only with an error in following principles or with an artificial illusion that imitates them. Hence there is a natural and unavoidable dialectic of pure reason, not one in which a bungler might be entangled through lack of acquaintance, or one that some sophist has artfully invented in order to confuse rational people, but one that irremediably attaches to human reason, so that even after we have exposed the mirage it will still not cease to lead our reason on with false hopes, continually propelling it into momentary aberrations that always need to be removed.[5]

I would like to emphasize from this passage Kant's awareness of the unavoidability of the illusion ensuing from the structures of reason. Everything in his analysis hints at the fact that the human mind can just prepare itself for encountering mirages unable to be cleared up through a neat explanation of the chain of mistakes committed. Put it slightly differently: Kant's approach to reason considers that this faculty tends to deviate understanding and judgement from the normative use of their operations. Yet to be wary of the pernicious effects stemming from the paradoxical "rational illusion" does not entail to discard any contribution deriving from this faculty to epistemic progress. On the contrary, Kant affirms in the *Transcendental Dialectic* of the first *Critique* that the ideas of pure reason need to be used in a non-deceptive way, which consists in expanding the perspective that the subject has over the cognitive field:

> The ideas of pure reason can never be dialectical in themselves; rather it is merely their misuse which brings it about that a deceptive illusion

> arises out of them; for they are given as problems for us by the nature of our reason, and this highest court of appeals for all rights and claims of our speculation cannot possibly contain original deceptions and semblances. Presumably, therefore, they have their good and purposive vocation in regard to the natural predisposition of our reason.[6]

As is well known, the court of reason has to sort out the rightful claims and groundless pretentions of human mental faculties,[7] while acknowledging the support that ideas of reason may furnish for giving the knowledge a systematic shape. As one reads in a lecture on metaphysics from the mid-1770s, this cooperation between understanding and reason allows that "[t]he understanding does not go beyond the boundaries of the objects of the senses, but still up to the boundary: this is God and the future world" (V-MetL1: 28:240). This interaction among human faculties entails some changes in the division usually projected over the rational and irrational actions in the human mind,[8] as it is a matter of fact that reason inspires a set of unavoidable illusions, which from a certain standpoint might foster the extension of possible knowledge. As some interpreters have stressed, that reason is naturally devoted to metaphysics opens up a long gallery of illusions,[9] which the transcendental philosopher should exhaustively be acquainted with. Notwithstanding this fact, Kant seems to be convinced that a little bit of madness could be advisable to enliven the common sense of the human mind. If neglecting the danger it has to face as it dives into metaphysical issues, the subject becomes more vulnerable in the epistemic field as it is usually. As Kant underscores in his published anthropology book, the popular claims uttering that someone "has crossed the line" or "the equator for the first time" (Anth 7: 218), as felicitous sentences to express the physical movement underpinning mental disorder deserve an accurate meditation about the correlate between madness and the consciousness of the space which the human being can view and control.

The Rules of Madness in Kant's Pragmatic Anthropology

Kant's approach to mental illness follows a systematic thread, for displaying the forms of disorder that human nature may develop and give in inheritance to its descendants. According to the logical scheme that Kant follows, anthropological exploration admits two species of mental disturbance, that is, *melancholia* or *hypochondria*, widely explored throughout cultural history, and *mental derangement*.[10] Even if the first one does not properly belong to the forms of derangement, it might be considered as a sort of threshold of the disordered functioning of the human faculties. The hypochondriac subject cannot help developing a silly anxiety corresponding to the inner physical sensations he receives from the external world.

Thus the mind obsessively concentrates its attention in the inner reflection related to some "local impressions", as the unease ensuing after a meal or dinner, figuring a "physical disease" stemming from a "real physical ailment" (Anth 7: 212).[11] Put differently, the hypochondriac used to appear in the European culture as an imaginarily ill person, who undergoes a sort of child regression, which urges the doctors to prescribe him placebos to calm down the anxiety the subject himself brings about. Moreover, another feature of hypochondriac people induces them to read medicine books and believe that they suffer from all the ailments they describe. Kant stresses the fact that this form of life makes the subject incapable for happiness, as he himself fosters the causes that hinder him to attain any real and enduring satisfaction. Therefore, this subject confounds the real with the imaginary and becomes the worst enemy of the pleasures he might feel in contact with life. Just the capacity of abstraction may in Kant's view wane the pernicious effects of the classical disposition to *melancholia*, insofar as it distracts the subject from this strenuous activity and forces him to heed to objective phenomena around him.[12]

Yet a manifold disability to build a coherent experience and to behave as a responsible person characterizes mental derangement, which according to Kant requires a deep engagement from philosophers and the philosophy faculty, as he deems the physicians and psychologists not trained for shedding light, for example, on the responsibility or innocence of people who commit crimes as they suffer the physical disease of madness.[13] In this context it is quite shocking Kant's concern about the tendency to view most criminals as insane people, "people whom we should pity and cure, but not punish" (Anth.: 7: 214, footnote), as this account forestalls to dispense legal justice.

Kant concretely hints at the case of a woman having committed infanticide because she had been sentenced to be locked into a penitentiary and deemed that this fate was worse than death. The judge charged with the case exempted her from the death penalty, yielding as argument that her mind was insane as she executed the murder of her child.

Considering the way Kant argues about this case, if the courts would begin to apply this line of argumentation in their sentences, this would deeply compromise the handing down of a sound notion of justice to subsequent generations. Even if the traits Kant attributes for instance to *Wahnsinn*, that is, *dementia*, are close to what contemporary psychiatry views as a paranoid character,[14] it is a key point in his account the claim of the legal responsibility of insane people, insofar as he views all human beings, independently of their mental health condition, as provided with human dignity and ethical accountability. Moreover, a philosophical theory of mental illness should not endanger the universal application of Kant's ethics and the notion of freedom it unfolds. Yet to endorse an excessively tender and merciful account of mental disorder would appear as a sort of blind spot able to ruin the value of moral responsibility. At any rate, the most original point in Kant's approach to delirious people highlights the expertise that philosophers would have with regard to the disturbed mind, surpassing by far the analytical acuteness of psychologists and physicians, who limit their knowledge of the human body to a material survey.[15]

With regard to mental disorder, Kant does not hesitate to call it the "most profound degradation of humanity" (Anth 7: 214), stemming from a crooked nature inherited through generations.[16] The pragmatic account of mental illness highlights the fact that the patients do not cooperate for retrieving their mental health, as the disorder of their mental faculties hinders any fruitful therapy. Mental frailties are kept out from this approach, as they are not so harmful as mental illness.[17] Yet Kant breaks down different sorts of these incurable disorders, following the thread of the dynamics that mental powers engage with each other and sketching an evolutive overview, which goes from the less severe illness to the gravest one. Thus, the philosopher distinguishes between *amentia* (*Unsinnigkeit*), *dementia* (*Wahnsinn*), *insania* (*Wahnwitz*) and *vesania* (*Aberwitz*). Each of these disorders displays in turn a tumultuous, methodical, fragmentary and systematic disproportion between powers such as perception, imagination and judgement. *Amentia* stems from the incapacity to build up with perceptions a coherent experience for the action of an excessive and boisterous imagination, which prevents the establishing of any comprehensible ties between the discourse of the lunatic person and the phenomena she intends to hint at (Anth 7: 214–215). As a second sort of disturbance, *dementia* appears when the subject seems to be able to meet the formal rules of possible experience. Yet a too inventive imagination turns "self-made representations" into perceptions of real facts.[18] This kind of mentally ill person reminds one of the persecutory manic, who suffers from a hidden narcissism that ruins any social life:

> Those who believe that they are surrounded by enemies everywhere, who consider all glances, words, and otherwise indifferent actions of others as aimed against them personally and as traps set for them, belong in this category. – In their unhappy delusion they are often so astute in interpreting that which others do naturally as aimed against them that, if only the data were true, we would have to pay due honor to their understanding.
>
> (Anth 7: 215)

In this passage, Kant focuses on the destructive character that demented people represent for themselves. The case of lunacy depicted in the passage might be hinting at the neurotic disturbance that the French philosopher Rousseau suffered all his life, even employing this endemic ailment as material for developing his claims about the human condition. For this reason, they do not deserve to be locked in asylums – some of them become well-known intellectuals, notwithstanding Kant's epistemic blindness towards this fact – as they are actually the worst enemy for themselves. Their obsession with inner derangements appears as the fastest path to unhappiness, leaving aside any external context provoking depression. Kant also hints at the fact that the use of drugs might incline the subject to develop *dementia*, as these substances introduce disorder in the feeling about the activity of the mind. Thus, the Flemish physician Helmont had the impression he may think with his stomach after tasting a dose of wolfsbane root and people experimenting with opium tend to fall into mental deficiency after long use (Anth 7: 216–217). Drug abuse leads thus easily to a disability to control human faculties. A third species of mental disorder leads to *insania*, which Kant qualifies as "deranged *power of judgment*" (Anth 7: 215), where imagination plays to supersede the role that understanding fulfils in weaving experience.[19] Here the outlandish analogies attempt to outshine the function of concepts, giving shape to a sort of creative and entertaining lunatic who tends to write bad poetry. Moreover, the illusion of experience stemming from this mental illness just offers a fragmentary overview of the mental chimeras ingrained in the lunatic mind. Finally, the last species of mental derangement – *vesania* – discloses a kind of "positive unreason" (Anth 7: 216), which makes the subject believe in being able to display an alternative experience, where the laws of the unknown would be revealed to the patient. Thus, impossible issues of knowledge, as the squaring of the circle, perpetual motion, the unveiling of the supersensible or the explanation of the Holy Trinity, appear as topics that the patient purports to be acquainted with, and furthermore available to be shared with ordinary people. Kant stresses the systematic style of the "self-enclosed speculation" typical in this kind of lunatic, which allows one to see them as "the calmest of all hospital patients" (Anth 7: 216).[20] This approach also highlights the fact that the mind of the vesanic subject seems to inhabit another world different from the one shared by human beings, far away from common sense. Moreover, these lunatics undergo a derangement (*Verrückung*) of the mind that completely changes the view they have about the phenomena they consider real, "just as a mountainous landscape sketched from a bird's-eye view prompts a completely different judgment about the region that when is viewed from the level ground" (Anth 7: 216). Thus, this sort of extreme mental disorder sets out an astonishing phenomenon, as it confirms that even the most disturbed animal life in human beings still needs "a principle of unity" to have the delusional impression that at least the subject *thinks* to a certain degree.

All forms of madness exhibit that the subjects suffering from the mentioned diseases have lost the *common sense*, which they have replaced by a *private sense* that isolates them into an imaginary world (Anth 7: 219), where they believe to see and hear phenomena that other human beings cannot grasp. Put slightly differently, mad people live in "[their] own world (as in dreaming)", made of "a play of thoughts" (Anth 7: 219) they loosely sketch. They should not be confounded with trailblazing poets, who explore human imagination for retrieving quaint analogies and metaphors.[21] Thus, it will not be surprising to ascertain that madness as mental derangement spoils the disciplinary role that the understanding of others has in the developmental process of the human mind. In fact, Kant highlights that social intercourse might suppose a therapy to prevent mental disorder, even if it does not help when hereditary ailments or drug abuse plunge the subject into the abyss of derangement. It is also interesting to pay attention to the fact that even if species of madness might recall traits close to childish behavior, Kant stresses that there are no mad children, as this disorder only buds with the development of reason.[22]

Kant's Approach to Social Life as Inhibitor of Mental Illness

Kant's analysis of mental illness reveals that mental isolation fosters disorder in the normative interaction among the faculties of the mind. Moreover, the egoism that mental derangement entails makes the subject plunge into a labyrinth of delusory fears and expectations. In this context, to get acquainted with cultural activities might fulfil a therapeutic role for the subject exposed to the risks of a melancholic temperament, for instance.[23] Thus, hypochondria invites to contravene the rules helping weave a coherent experience, insofar as this mental attitude invites the subject to excessively inspect her inner representations, losing any correlation with the judgement of others. A large text archive stemming from the *Lectures on Anthropology* confirms this view about the melancholic temperament and character:

> Thus, for instance, hypochondriac subjects constantly pay attention to themselves, and since they use to view themselves as an object, they also display often absurd claims in society, which draws the attention of "ordinary people", who meet the requirements of social normativity. All this feeling of oneself is actually counterproductive. For what I feel is of no use. The more information one has about objects, however, the more useful one is. With an ever-present feeling of oneself, one loses one's entire activity and liveliness, the human being becomes a true dreamer, because his imagination, which is not led by his understanding, produces all sorts of chimaeras and the worst moods and follies.

> Withdrawal from this self-feeling is an elevation of the mind, which is effected if I let my mind roam into different representations through a voluntary distraction in society. By which ceases the attention to oneself. A healthy soul is always concerned with something outside itself.[24]

Subjected to the hegemony of a powerful inner sense activity, the melancholic subject fails to draw to his power to abstract to open up an exit from mental illness. As previously said, Kant trusts very much the capacity of social distraction to retrieve the subject from the excesses of lunacy, which actually requires that he grasps the ordinary delusions circulating through the social realm.[25] Thus, our author upholds that to enter into a society requires that the subject got previously acquainted with the art of deceit admissible in the social spaces. Different reasons explain how "moral illusion" and the "virtues of social intercourse" boost social ties and help escape from mental disorder. With regard to the first phenomenon – moral illusion – Kant does not hesitate to recognize that human beings behave as actors inasmuch as they engage in the civilized condition. Yet this disposition to act in public before others does not mean any moral stain. Quite on the contrary, people having adopted the use of affection, respect or modesty as a mere illusion towards others become ready to act according with these values. Put slightly differently, the subject who adopts this behavior achieves "to deceive the deceiver" (Anth 7: 151), which in the case of the human being hints at the inclinations and the overview of happiness they promise. For fleshing out the content of this action, Kant retrieves an eloquent sentence from Jonathan Swift's writings, which urges to "surrender a barrel for the whale to play with, in order to save the ship" (Anth 7: 152). The process reminds the well-known coaching motto "fake it till do it" and fulfils a key role in Kant's practical philosophy. Thus, Kant positively assesses the "tendency ... to be deceived" (Anth 7: 152), which is related to the cultural phenomenon called *decorum* by the Latins, whose heir in Kant's time would be politeness – the successful French *politesse*, which all European royal courts claim as an identity sign – defined as "an illusion of affability that inspires love" (Anth 7: 152). Moreover, he argues for the positive effect ensuing from social deceit as it finally fosters the adoption of a moral character:

> It is only the illusion of good *in ourselves* that must be wiped out without exception, and the veil by which self-love conceals our moral defects must be torn away. For illusion does *deceive*, if one deludes oneself that one's debt is cancelled or even thrown away by that which is without any moral content, or persuades oneself that one is not guilty —e.g., when repentance for misdeeds at the end of one's life is depicted as real improvement, or intentional transgressions as human weakness.[26]

Leaving aside the negative impact on morality stemming from the illusion about the good deeds the subject carries out, Kant recommends to cultivate social virtues (*virtutes homileticae*) (MM 6: 473), as they are expected to help us cultivate our moral perfection in social intercourse with other human beings not suspicious of living in outrageous vice.[27] According with this account, insofar as people behave showing respect, tolerance, agreeableness and mutual love to other, a disposition of reciprocity buds in the hearts. Thus, a sort of by-products (*parerga*) of virtue provide a kind of non-deceptive illusion of virtue,[28] as everybody knows that a general knowledge about the value of affability, sociability, courtesy and hospitality as mere tokens undergirds their use. Kant stresses the point that these quasi-virtues "bring ... illusion as near as possible to the truth" (MM 6: 473–474). Dinner parties, which Kant considers "the highest ethicophysical good", play a key role in this contribution that social enjoyment makes to morality, in taking strong roots in human nature. The combination of a good conversation with moderate amounts of tasty food hints thus to the very gist of the human condition, which intertwines physical needs with moral tasks. Kant stresses the good-natured function that borders fulfil as people eat and drink together, underscoring that "to go a bit beyond the borderline of sobriety for a short while" (Anth 7: 171) belongs to the mum covenant that gives birth to social life. Naturally, Kant does not endorse a naïve approach to human nature, but he rather claims that to keep back one's own beliefs and arguments might be a prudent conduct compared to a too open-hearted attitude, which should be better endorsed in the context of a public dinner party.[29] It is worthwhile to remember at this point a passage where Kant sketches the model of coexistence of rational beings who were not able to think but aloud:

> It could well be that on some other planet there might be rational beings who could not think in any other way but aloud; that is, they could not have any thoughts that they did not at the same time *utter*, whether awake or dreaming, in the company of others or alone. What kind of behavior toward others would this produce, and how would it differ from that of our human species? Unless they were all *pure angels*, it is inconceivable how they could live in peace together, how anyone could have any respect at all for anyone else, and how they could get on well together.[30]

The form of life of these beings stands out for the close points it shows to have in common with regard to mental illness. In fact, some lunatic subjects cannot avoid expressing what they think loudly, which should not be considered an instance of sharing thought and beliefs, but rather as a sign of human egoism and mental isolation. Put differently, Kant's example about the form of life of other imaginary rational beings helps make us more aware of the benefits ensuing from withholding our own impressions and judgements about some issues, especially those that might unnecessarily expose our social respect and status. Even if social life is helpless towards the total removal of mental illnesses from humanity, which Kant deems impossible to endeavor, it can discourage the emergence of such disturbances as they depend on forms of life the subject wrongly engages in, insofar as social intercourse trains human imagination and simultaneously maintains it under control.

Concluding Remarks

Throughout this chapter, I attempted to claim that Kant's account of mental illness shares key traits with the critical project. Given this, the establishment of sound boundaries determining which is cognizable or not for human beings fulfils the goals of transcendental philosophy, which intends to display an accurate geography of the faculties of the mind. Moreover, the subject who overviews from his standpoint a space extended beyond boundaries that were rightly set may be deceived by it, insofar as he confuses the immanent use the critique admits of it with a transcendent one, which leads the human mind to a barren field of delusions. Just when the critical method highlights the regulative use of transcendent structures as ideas of reason, the subject discovers he may draw on them to enlarge the view and scope of the knowledge he attains. As Kant's interpreters have claimed since decades, madness belongs to the very gist of reason as a potential development of it. Yet the task to make of *common sense* a hegemonic attitude in the human community nourishes the hope to lessen the effects ensuing from mental disturbance. Furthermore, anthropological analysis comes to give support to the aims of critique as a mental therapy, as it highlights the advantages that the social value of appearance guarantees to the human mind. Moreover, as I attempted to address above, Kant does not discard appearance as a deceitful dispositive that should be banned from the moral development of human beings. On the contrary, to engage in a sort of social play, which helps people get acquainted with the formal requirements of a peaceful society, committed to fulfil the sundry duties of aid and respect of others, will progressively give shape to a sounder society.

Even if mental illness condemns the subject to isolation, as the mad subject lacks any means to communicate his thoughts to others, to inspect its forms contributes to strengthen the awareness that the epistemic normative subject has of the sources of weakness and frailty of the mind. Kant addresses social intercourse as a space working on driving away mental disorder, even if the maze of appearances embedded in society may also have a negative impact on the subject, making him distrustful and conspiranoid, as Rousseau claimed in some of his writings. At least the set of humanity not touched by the stain of inherited mental illness may engage in social intercourse as an opportunity to train his epistemic and moral faculties, getting used to take into account the standpoint of others as he performs his cognitive and practical tasks. Notwithstanding the neutral value Kant assigns to *common sense*, which nominally should overlap all potential individual standpoints and fulfil the role of an ideal for all of them, the interpreter might claim that social discipline frames human capacities, adapting them to social imagination. Put differently, just the genial poet or artist goes around as an accepted exception through the social space, without any fear to be locked in a lunatic asylum, as their genial images and appearances challenge the common sense, but at the same time strengthen it. Yet unlike the excessive imagination of the genial artist, lunatic people do not notice any difference between reality and fiction. Thus, they become non-yielding passive social agents, a category stemming from Kant's anthropological writings that deserves further exploration, as it hints to the blind spots of Kant's practical philosophy, which once and again claims that not all human beings would deserve to be treated as worthy of the humanity they materially embody.

Notes

1 See also the distinction between *appearance* (*Erscheinung*) and *illusion* (*Schein*) in R 4999 (1776–78, 18:56). Kant's writings are quoted according to the volume and page number of the *Akademie Ausgabe*, I. Kant, *Gesammelte Schriften*, previously Königlich-Preussische, now Deutsche Akademie der Wissenschaften, Berlin, 1900 – and following the abbreviation of the *Kant-Forschungsstelle* of the University of Mainz. For the English translations of Kant's writings, I follow the Cambridge Edition of *Works of Immanuel Kant*.

2 Prol. 4: 352. See also Howard 2022 and Constantini 2021: 104: "the critical Kant has preferred the 'Grenze', the limit of space, to the 'Limitation', the limit of reality, and to him madness, especially that of reason, takes on the appearance of the overcoming of a line drawn before one's eye, since it is perceived within a precise geometry of the psychic space. Such geometry has all the appearance of being designed for the purpose of limiting imagination on multiple sides, thereby preventing it from any form of excess – creating, de facto, the conditions for an excess, in general, to occur".

3 About this epistemic unacceptable barter, which takes something subjective for objective, see Anth 7: 114.

4 KrV A 235–236/B 294–295.

5 KrV, A 297/298-B 354–355. Cfr. KrV A339/B 397: "They are sophistries not of human beings but of pure reason itself, and even the wisest of all human beings cannot get free of them; perhaps after much effort he may guard himself from error, but he can never be wholly rid of the illusion, which ceaselessly teases and mocks him". See also Feloj (2021: 314).

6 KrV A 669/B 697.

7 See Møller (2020: 17–19).

8 See Feloj 2021: 319: "If one accepts transcendental illusion as inevitable, and if one agrees with the idea that the doctrine of illusion provides the foundation to errors of judgment and even insanity, then Kant seems to be decisively eschewing the opposition between rational and irrational. Illusion, error, and even insanity are included in the very definition of the use of reason. However, this does not mean, as Foucault (2009) claimed, that the Enlightenment advocates a submission of madness to reason according to a process of assimilation to mental illness".

9 See for instance Jalley-Crampe 1979: 12 "reason unfolds [a hyperactivity] when it dreams whilst being awake or, which is the same thing, when it's devoted to metaphysics".

10 See Anth 7: 212 and V-Anth/Mron 25: 1302–1303: "Genuine mental illness concerns merely the state of the mind, the wrong use of the powers, even if in themselves they are good. Mental illness includes hypochondria, [and] considered from the perspective of the mind, melancholia".

11 In the *Investigation Concerning Diseases of the Head* Kant affirms that "[t]he chimeras which this illness hatches do not properly deceive our senses, but rather only make for the hypochondriac an illusion of the experience of his own state, either of the body or the soul, that is largely a mere crochet [*Grille*]". See the remarks of Meld Shell 1996: 268–269 and 284–285.

12 About the role that attention fulfils in Kant's account of mental disorder see Fleitas 2022: 302–303: "what is often not found in Kant's account of mental weaknesses and illnesses is the underlying role that attention plays. He specifically notes that a peculiar trait of these mental conditions is to hinder our mastery of the direction of our ideas, experiences, and decisions. Hypochondria as well as mania, i.e., the two types of dementia that Kant finds, are characterized for differentially partializing our control over the direction our mind takes, sometimes hyperfocusing our attention – hypochondria – other times seizing it by creating a rule that causes thought to be consistent with itself, but opposing the rules of the experience – mania. Kant seems to always relate the inability to master our attention to the inability to control our reason".

13 For instance, Kant disavows the attempt of Ernst Platner to dissect a human capacity as memory, breaking down nerves and fibers. According to the critical philosophy, a (logical, moral, aesthetical) function could not be reduced to an amount of material features, yet it requires to be grasped as a function. I focused on this issue in Sánchez Madrid (2018: 161–162).

14 See Constantini 2021: 100. See also the account of Silva (2019: 663): "*Dementia (Wahnsinnigkeit)* is perhaps the amplest of all the disturbances, and in it the lack of balance between powers focuses on the power of imagination, which in this state strives to realize fantasies; that is, it holds fantasies as real things. Namely, in it occurs a weak use of the senses, but possibly a good understanding and surely an exacerbated fantasy."

15 The whole § 51 of Anth (7: 213–214) stresses this epistemic privilege of philosophy compared to psychology and medicine on diagnosing mental disorder.

16 He just excerpts *dementia* from biological hereditary legacy. See V-Anth/Mron 25: 1288.

17 An account of Kant's distinction between mental frailty and mental illness might be drawn from Silva (2019: 662–663).

18 See also V-Anth/Fried, 25: 514: "If however the imagination is intense, then the intensity can also be excessive, so that the imagination often outweighs the sensible impression".

19 On the failure of understanding as the subject falls into lunacy see V-Anth/Fried 25: 544: "The sickness of the understanding consists either in lack of understanding, and this is stupidity, or in its being upside down, and this is insanity, or lunacy".

20 In the case of mad people who conduct themselves with fury, which makes the subject completely blunt to any external sensation, Kant urges physicians to apply the medicines more helpful to remove the material causes of the derangement. It is quite curious also in this text the epistemic authority that the philosopher intends to have towards the physician, as the expertise of the first one appears as more valuable to diagnose when the ailed body needs to receive medical substances.

21 Some interpreters have correctly highlighted the subtle boundaries between *genius* and *madness*, poetical fantasy and *dementia*, which will become a philosophical topos in Kant's account. A recent interpretation of this issue is Silva (2019: 679): "the demented, seized by the *sensus proprius* of his understanding, produces untruthful, even absurd representations, whereas in the poet the special disposition of his powers, along with the *sensus communis*, renders his images truthful and hence universally communicable and understandable. The poet, one could say, passes off as a man of follies but in him, and in his controlled irrationality, the images end up composing the ground of active humanity". I fully agree with Silva's claim, which makes of the use of understanding and its disposition to *sensus communis* the watershed point for acknowledging when the subject proceeds genially or simply as a lunatic.

22 See V-Anth/Fried 25: 528–529: "Madness or delirium is habitual fantasizing, thus taking the images for actual external objects. Who takes his chimera for actual objects of his previous state, for example, he was to have been a prince, is mad. However, who believes he sees external objects, is insane; both are delirium. Mad children do not exist, rather madness arises with reason. Madness due to illness is fantasizing or babbling".

23 See Feloj 2021: 131: "[I]n Kant's treatment of melancholy, cultivating culture and fine arts becomes a duty towards oneself, a duty that according to his philosophical dietetics allows the melancholic tendency to deep thoughts and prevents against the melancholic state of boredom".

24 V-Anthr/Bu 25: 1438–1439.

25 Kant recommends to engage in social intercourse for healing from the pernicious effects of melancholy in V-Anthr/Fried 25: 489: "When hypochondriacs have heard or seen something, it always keeps running through their heads and plagues them constantly, for example if they are present at an execution. One need not fear that they will also commit a wrongdoing, rather it is the failing of their power of choice, which does not have the power to abstract".

26 Anth 7: 153.

27 Cohen has accurately teased out this dimension of social illusion, see specially Cohen (2008: 318–320).

28 I previously focused on this issue in Kant's anthropology in Sánchez Madrid (2015: 129–137).

29 For getting an overview of this dependence of human nature on social appearances, see MM 6: 472.

30 Anth 7: 332.

References

Cohen, Alix, "The Ultimate Kantian Experience: Kant on Dinner Parties". *History of Philosophy Quarterly* 25, no. 4 (2008): 315–336.

Constantini, Marco, "Madness in the Organic Order of Space. Madness and Imagination". *Con-textos Kantianos* 13 (2021): 97–113.

Feloj, Serena, "Kant on Melancholy: Philosophy as a Relief to the Disgust of Life". *Con-textos Kantianos* 13 (2021): 123–132.

Fleitas, Martín, "A Kantian Sovereignty of Attention as a Therapy for Mental Illnesses". *Con-textos Kantianos. International Journal of Philosophy* 15 (2022): 297–310.

Foucault, M., *History of Madness*. Edited by J. Khalfa and J. Murphy. London: Routledge, 2009.

Howard, Stephen, "Kant on Limits, Boundaries, and the Positive Function of Ideas". *European Journal of Philosophy* 30 (2022): 64–78.

Jalley-Crampe, M., "La raison et ses rêves. Kant juge de Swedenborg". *Revue des sciences humaines* 176 (1979): 9–21.

Meld Shell, Susan, *The Embodiment of Reason. Kant on Spirit, Generation, and Community*. Chicago/London: University of Chicago Press, 1996.

Møller, Sophie, *Kant's Tribunal of Reason: Legal Metaphor and Normativity in the Critique of Pure Reason*. Oxford: Oxford University Press, 2020.

Sánchez Madrid, Nuria, "Controlling Mental Disorder: Kant's Account of Mental Illness in the Anthropology Writings". In G. Lorini, and R.B. Louden (eds.), *Knowledge, Morals and Practice in Kant's Anthropology*. Cham: Palgrave Macmillan, 2018, pp. 147–162.

Sánchez Madrid, Nuria, "La profondeur des dispositifs civilisateurs: la dialectique negative entre la politesse et la moralité chez l'anthropologie de Kant". *ÉNDOXA: Series Filosóficas* 35 (2015): 119–138.

Silva, Fernando, "'Dementia is a fiction'. Kant on the Mental Disturbances of the Human Soul". *Tijdschrift voor Filosofie* 81 (2019): 657–680.

3 The Madness of Guilt

Against Contemporary Approaches to Shame and Guilt

Ana Falcato

Introduction

In *The Greeks and the Irrational* (Dodds, 1951), Eric Dodds begins his exposition of the Greek mindset by recounting an experience from everyday life – a casual visit to the British Museum, during which a fellow tourist commented upon the *rationalistic* worldview of the ancient Greeks, a spiritual feature to which Greek statuary bears witness. Throughout the book, he then unfolds a systematic argument against the tourist's aesthetic intuition by unearthing some of the most impressive manifestations of the *irrational* in Greek thought and myth.

The Greeks and the Irrational is an impressive example of classical Greek scholarship, and I do not aim to discuss its exquisite historical and philological portrait of the Greek mindset in detail here. Instead, I aim to isolate a structural account of both irrational guilt-mechanisms and their genetic development, which can speculatively be traced either to a historic-religious source (as Dodds does) or, more prosaically, to individual psychogenetic roots. Building on the main insights of Dodds's masterpiece regarding this specific emotional pattern, I aim in this chapter to situate them in a cultural setting more akin to our own – a twenty-first century global context – and to explain what can be not only irrational but *maddening* about guilt and guilt-mechanisms.

To accomplish this – thus confirming Dodds's most important insight while following a strictly secular argumentative path – I will: (1) extract the details of the moral argument behind Dodds's presentation of the genesis of guilt-mechanisms in cultures with a religious frame of mind, like that of the ancient Greeks; (2) adapt and refine this interpretive model to match secular notions of both guilt and shame; and (3) describe certain flaws in the most convincing contemporary moral attacks on guilt and guilt-mechanisms, in light of the model defended by Dodds. In doing so, I will confirm the accuracy of Dodds's structural insight concerning guilt and guilt-mechanisms: the idea that guilt as a cultural phenomenon

DOI: 10.4324/9781003288992-5

will either overwhelm the subject and lead to self-destruction or rescue her from a self-inflicted moral abyss.

Shame- and Guilt-Cultures

In his 1949 Sather Classical Lectures, Eric Dodds had an extremely complex conceptual story to tell about the transition from a so-called shame-culture to a so-called guilt-culture in the Archaic period – a story that has often been misrepresented or simplified even in competent contemporary scholarship on these anthropological notions (see Williams, 1993).[1] Its basic – and structural – insight runs as follows: The Archaic age (roughly, the period between the eighth century BCE and the first decades of the fifth century BCE) witnessed the growth of the Greek economy and an expansion of its imperial might in the Atlantic, the immediate cultural impact of which was a deep sense, on the part of the Greeks, of the perils of collective *hybris* and success and a fear of warranted retribution by the gods. This sense of *endangered glory* would go on to foster a modular guilt response in which the disparity between human frailty and ambition, on the one hand, and divine power, on the other, was paramount. It also explained the strong guilt response on the part of the human agent who was subject to the wrath of a mighty divinity.

Without getting into the complex philological details of Dodds's hermeneutic model, I would like to approach his account from the standpoint of a philosophical investigation into shame and guilt, tracing its main argumentative steps. One fundamental insight from this lecture (titled 'From Shame-Culture to Guilt-Culture') is that the tragic poets – especially Sophocles and Euripides – established a sort of axiological break with the Homeric tradition, mapping out a new social order from which religious elements were never absent.

Likely at the time of Solon[2] (explicit reference to Solon's laws is never made in the text, but his name is mentioned several times, and his dates are a match for Dodds's hypothesis), social relations in mainland Greece were deeply rooted in the family, and the figure of the father functioned, both literally and symbolically, as a moral authority. Fear of the wrath of the gods and of paternal punishment worked in tandem, forming a central feature of the kind of irrationality at stake in the second lecture of *The Greeks and the Irrational*.

Dodds analyses this socio-cultural pattern of behavior in light of the notion of divine *pthónos*, a Greek word that he translates as 'jealousy'. Thus, in what is likely the most relevant passage in the book when it comes to the personal dynamics of self-blaming, we read the following:

> The proverbial saying popular in that age that 'all virtue is comprehended in justice', applies no less to gods than to men: there was little

> room for pity in either. ... But in becoming the embodiment of cosmic justice, Zeus lost his humanity. Hence Olympianism in its moralized form tended to become a religion of fear, a tendency which is reflected in the religious vocabulary.
>
> (Dodds, 1951: 35)

It is worth noting that Dodds is here – and indeed throughout the entire study – focusing his analysis on examples of irrationality in the Greek *Weltanschauung* that had an expressive impact on the literary repository of the culture as a whole and that can be used to construct a psychological model. In this chapter, his analytical target is the formation of a personal (and cosmological) *feeling of guilt*.

Dodds ventures the hypothesis that it was because of the pervasiveness of the Olympian religion in the collective life of a culture threatened from the outside by war and (minimally) connected from the inside by ancient family bonds – all while the individual was incentivized to thrive and lead a life of prestige – that social portraits of guilt became conspicuous in Archaic Greece. On Dodds's account, this genealogical structure justifies for the aura of guilt that pervaded Greek society as a whole.

Two things immediately stand out in this regard. One is the connection between the cosmic element of this emotional pattern and its singular manifestations in each individual; the other is the relevance of this social, historically situated *Erlebnis* to the characteristic elements of an ethical experience we all recognise. It will strike the casual reader that Dodds must be either exaggerating the terms of his analysis when depicting the spiritual features of guilt or discussing a culture that is so far removed from our own that it is puzzling how the latter could have been viewed as one of its spiritual predecessors. What I mean by this structural discrepancy (analysing feelings of guilt in terms of divine wrath) is that experiences of guilt do not usually depend on fear of divine *pthnónos* or of a disproportionate calamity, far beyond the resources of the human being, in order to manifest themselves in one's life.

When one looks more closely at the details of Dodds's analysis of the formation of guilt in terms of the ancient mindset, however, neither of the two options holds true – that is, neither is this a model of an *alien* cultural framework, nor is the general picture an exaggerated one. When Dodds completes his 'cultural diagnostic' of the transition from a 'shame-culture' to a 'guilt-culture', drawing on several sources from Greek myth, poetry and even philosophy (the last 'evidence' for his thesis is Plato's handling of the story of Oedipus in the *Republic*), the most conspicuous scientific support for this cultural shift is ultimately Freudian psychoanalysis (see Dodds, 1951: 47–48). In fact, throughout the several lectures that make up the book, the constant aim is to bring Greek sources as close as possible to contemporary psychological models. Thus, the explanation of the constitution of guilt-feelings, according to Dodds, is completely modern; only the textual material to which it is applied is not. On the other hand, one must be very careful about our own 'secularized' reading of this (doubly classic, i.e., epistemically and historically) diagnostic of guilt-feelings, especially when it is contextualized as a model to account for a *cultural shift*. What this means is that Dodds's framework for understanding an emotional response that we also thematize in the context of secular societies and in 'post-religious' cultures may bear more resemblance to what we today experience as feelings of guilt than may first appear.

Here is how Dodds concludes his examination of a moral outlook based on guilt – an account based in part on his reading of Archaic poetry:

> You see perhaps where all this is tending. The psychologists have taught us how potent a source of guilt-feelings is the pressure of unacknowledged desires, desires which are excluded from consciousness save in dreams or daydreams, yet are able to produce in the self a deep sense of moral uneasiness. This uneasiness often takes a religious form today; and if a similar feeling existed in Archaic Greece, this would be the natural form for it to take. For, to begin with, the human father had from the earliest times his heavenly counterpart; *Zeus pater* belongs to the Indo-European inheritance, as his Latin and Sanskrit equivalents indicate; ... In cult also Zeus appears as a supernatural Head of the Household; ... It was natural to project on to the heavenly Father those curious mixed feelings which the child dared not acknowledge even to himself.
>
> (Dodds, 1951: 48)

The organizing principle of this shift is straightforward: The patriarchal structure of a deeply religious society emulates in its cult the working mechanism of the family. What is astonishing about Dodds's proposal – especially when contrasted with certain modern and contemporary renderings of morality and moral feelings, including those developed by one of his brightest pupils, Bernard Williams[3] – is the fact that the charge of *irrationality* falls on the side of *guilt* rather than *shame*. The irrational moral response, in light of this genetic reading of the dawn of a primary moral feeling, is the guilty rather than the shameful one.

Dodds's lectures themselves must be put into context – and this in many ways. What he is tracing in them are setbacks in the evolution of Greek rationalism, from Homer to the tradition of Neoplatonism, of which *this shift* – from a shame-culture to a guilt-culture, from Homeric to Archaic society – is but one among many. At the same time, he is hinting at the ideological monsters of his own time (one must remember that these were the Sather Lectures of 1949) and warning against the temptation to patriarchal idolatry.

The more stable *nuances* of this borrowed psychological model, however, are perhaps worth mentioning, if only to stress how *reasonable* they in fact are – by which I mean how well we can make sense of the uneasiness characteristic of the mental mechanism sketched in these lectures, even in a social and moral context as far removed from that of sixth-century BCE mainland Greece as our own. If we consider the typically *sudden* and *transitory* aspects of delirium[4] (as clinically and etymologically defined) and link *guilt* to a form of *transition from one mode of self-apprehension to a different, more inclusive one in which a sense of personal wrongdoing makes one feel liable to punishment and seek immediate self-amendment*, then the exaggerated cosmic and burdensome features of this moral feeling (as presented in Dodds's analysis and in many other accounts of guilt as a moral emotion and a moral trigger)[5] all fall away, while the main psychological insights highlighted by the anthropological material here presented are preserved. Without at all wanting to force terminology or historical interpretations of terminological clusters, I would stress that what Dodds here takes to be *pools of irrational behavior* in the Greek rationalistic mindset might also be read as patterns of human behavior that are typically ungraspable by reason and thus by normal forms of conscious self-reflection. We simply do not realize that this kind of 'guilty homunculus' is something *we are* as well.

Experiencing guilt as a revealing episode of self-disclosure – which may formally manifest itself in the way Dodds describes it in the second lecture of *The Greeks and the Irrational* – may indeed feel like a maddening experience or an abrupt instantiation of a moral view with which we are all acquainted. We can experience guilt, as the Greeks did, as a thorough and *sudden* deviation from a familiar moral feeling and moral outlook that corresponds to our own most well-known character and moral persona – even in all its transitoriness and various manifestations – for 'moral character' is not a fixed set of moral features (like irremovable scars) but rather a nest of dispositions which vary with the inner and outer circumstances. However, and precisely because of the resonance of such an atypical form of moral shock[6] – that is, that of being caught in a crisis of profound personal guilt – the recovery effort may turn out to be akin to the sort of cathartic experience depicted in the verses from Sophocles' *Antigone* quoted at the end of the lecture:

> Blessed is he whose life has not tasted of evil.
> When God has shaken a house, the winds of madness
> Lash its breed till the breed is done:
> Even so the deep-sea swell
> Raked by wicked Thracian winds
> Scours in its running the subaqueous darkness,

Churns the silt black from sea-bottom;
And the windy cliffs roar as they take its shock. Here on the Labdacid
  house long we watched it piling,
Trouble on dead men's trouble: no generation
Frees the next from the stroke of God:
Deliverance does not come.[7]

As in Sophocles' *Antigone*, recovering from an episode of guilt may turn one's moral and mental life upside down and reshape one's core values and life path from that moment on – and this applies equally to non-tragic experiences of the emotion under analysis. I now turn to contemporary moral treatments of guilt and how they account – or fail to account – for this type of emotional crisis and deep personal conversion.

Guilt in Contemporary Moral Philosophy

According to the kind of cultural split presented above, the late transition from a shame-culture to a guilt-culture brought into being a mindset with more internalized and autonomous forms of response to wrongdoing and faults, and in both social and individual terms *guilt* then became the dominant moral feeling. A significant feature of the contemporary discussion of this pair of moral emotions – *shame* and *guilt* – is precisely our tendency to describe them in contrasting yet complementary terms. In the mid-twentieth-century anthropological literature, their structural features and moral predominance are described in order to account for cultural rifts, and in moral philosophy, their different phenomenologies are considered for the purpose of making metaethical decisions about which is worthier from a contemporary moral outlook.

The English philosopher Bernard Williams was particularly critical of the role played by *guilt* in the so-called Western modern moral outlook, and in his book *Shame and Necessity* he downplays the importance of guilt – specifically when contrasted with *shame* – in what he views as sane forms of moral behavior.[8] The target of his analysis is undoubtedly Kant – or at least contemporary readings of Kant[9] – and his definition of guilt and its impact on moral agents derives from a particular reading of the machinery of Kantian ethics – specifically Kant's notion of duty or moral obligation.

To begin with, Williams concentrates on providing a full-fledged definition of the experience of shame and defending its relevance to our moral lives.[10] Not only does his account of the phenomenology of guilt-feelings and their impact on one's moral predicament or emotional background play a less important role within the book's argument as a whole, but the main psychological features of the experience of guilt are sketchy on his reading, on the one hand, and also ancillary to his schematic portrait of the Kantian moral framework.

In contrast to the Kantian paradigm, the moral framework unearthed and praised by Bernard Williams was clearly downplayed by a generation of moral philosophers and classical scholars working within and defending the norm of the absolute *autonomy* of the moral agent. This normative paradigm is a widely acknowledged inheritance from Kantian practical philosophy, and it remains the main target of Williams's criticism throughout the whole of *Shame and Necessity*.

Perhaps the most acute criticism directed by Williams at contemporary advocates of Kantianism – also developed in his *Ethics and the Limits of Philosophy*[11] – is that modern readings of Kant's practical philosophy in which the structural moral significance of shame is rejected (in which shame, often stemming from involuntary action, is lumped together with a recognizable cluster of subjective responses that differ fundamentally from duty or action springing from sheer respect for the moral law) function unselfconsciously against the distorting background of the Kantian moral paradigm, which is taken as *given*. In other words, these readings project the Kantian norm of autonomy onto a specific classical ethical outlook; they assume, incongruently and anachronistically, that the main features of the Kantian moral subject are equally relevant to the classical framework. The result is a view according to which shame in Homeric culture is labeled and criticized as a *pre-* or *non-moral* experience.

Williams's critique of the moral context that privileges the absolute autonomy of the agent's will has two fundamental stages. Within the Kantian deontological framework, he claims, the autonomy of the moral agent is defined in terms of her immunity to the judgements of others in practical decision-making, that is, her ability to disregard such influences and instead act on principle. Autonomous freedom of choice is set against an adaptive model according to which each agent determines her actions with a view to meeting external expectations. Because the experience of shame is mainly connected with the disadvantageous exposure of oneself to the gaze of another, the values at stake are superficial, and superficial in a double sense. To the extent that the basic experience is related to the physical, to appearance, it concerns an appraisal of external features. For precisely this reason, the moral relevance of shame can be criticized: Shame does not concern the intrinsic value of the person and indeed replaces true value with what lies on the immediate surface – the first impression. If this were so, Williams continues (imagining the Kantian line of argument he wants to deconstruct), the experience of shame would indeed be linked to *heteronomy* and lack true moral value, since the self-directed adverse judgement involved in shame brings with it awareness of both the critical gaze of the other and how I appear in the light of that gaze, but nothing more.

On the other hand, and because the impression of disadvantage is merely subjective, the experience can be said to lack the universality that defines the Kantian normative model and could therefore be dismissed as *egoistic*. In fact, the two defining features tend to complement each other. An action is classified as egoistic if it is structurally motivated by the individual's desire for success and acclaim, and, it can be argued, such a practical pattern makes sense only given an environment in which the agent believes she will be seen and possibly receive acclaim. To be sure, agents can stipulate for themselves ends they would like to achieve, independently of third-party assessments or prescriptions. But even internalized expectations of personal fulfilment are learned and structured as patterns of self-assessment in the context of appearing in a world shared with others. What becomes in some sense *inner* – a part of my personal moral makeup, the backdrop against which I assess myself and my progress in the world – has its psychological roots at the level of my appearance among others. (Structurally, Williams argues, modern-day Kantian criticism levelled at the actions of the Archaic Greek hero can only sustain the balance of this double-edged attack by insisting on the *competitiveness* of the classical moral code – in a competition, any participant's aim is to win a contest the rules of which are accepted by all.)

However, and granted that the internalizing process is a widely acknowledged psychosocial fact, the mechanisms of shame are in fact neither strictly egoistic nor strictly heteronomous for Williams, but rather reside in a middle ground of internal self-assessment that is rooted in the psychological internalization of external standards of critical judgement. Interestingly, this deprives these mechanisms of *moralistic* connotations, whereby standardized norms of conduct are at once compulsory, made uniform and a-critically enacted.

This is Bernard Williams's brilliant treatment of a non-trivial experience of shame. But what, then, about *guilt* and its impact on one's ethical (or even existential) predicament? If one pays attention to Williams's criticism of Kant's moral paradigm, one sees that guilt is defined according to the double standard of *autonomy* and *universality*, and indeed as the negative – in terms of both worth and structural characteristics – of the (non-trivial) experience of shame. Consider, for instance, what Williams says about the contrast between the two emotions:

> We can see in terms of these models why shame might be thought to be in its very nature a more narcissistic emotion than guilt. The viewer's gaze draws the subject's attention not to the viewer, but to the subject himself; the victim's anger, on the other hand, draws attention to the victim. The suspicion of narcissism, I have argued in the text, can be overcome on the side of shame by widening one's view of its possible

> objects. ... But there is another consideration that should be borne in mind, on the side of guilt. If it is to be an inherent virtue of guilt, as opposed to shame, that it turns our attention to the victims of what we have wrongly done, then the victims and their feelings should remain figured in the construction of guilt, as they are in the primitive version of the model. When the conception of guilt is refined beyond a certain point and forgets its primitive materials of anger and fear, *guilt comes to be represented simply as the attitude of respect for an abstract law, and it then no longer has any special connection with victims.*[12] The victims may reenter, of course, in an account of what the subject has done in violation of that law, but that gives them, or thoughts of them, no more intimate connection to guilt than they have to shame. This is what I had in mind when I said earlier that the refinement of guilt in this direction can conceal one of its virtues.
>
> (Williams, 1993: 223)

As accurate as this description of the moral and psychological mechanisms at work in guilt-feelings may be, this is not the view of guilt as a moral and religious experience provided and criticized by Eric Dodds. Williams focuses his analysis on a refined – and textually unwarranted[13] – Kantian portrait of the experience of guilt, which is said to amount to the outcome of a violation of the moral law, and his criticism of the emotion does not contemplate any of the possible features of the experience highlighted by Dodds and expanded on in my comments above.

Williams is not interested in depicting guilt as a sudden, ethically damaging or even maddening experience that can turn one's core values and moral worldview upside down, prompting one to act on that feeling and *improve oneself* – other than in reference to what he claims to be wrong with the Kantian framework of duty and possible disrespect or disregard for moral duty.[14] This, however, was the extraordinary psychological and philological task taken up by Dodds – who, as astounding as it may sound from a Williamsian perspective, aligned himself with contemporary attempts to rehabilitate Greek views on ethical issues in modern moral life.[15]

Understanding the differences between Williams's specifically moral approach to this pair of negative moral emotions (and the kind of culture each of them helps to shape) and the alternative phenomenology of both emotional patterns that we find somewhat hidden within Dodds's analysis allows us to understand guilt in an altogether different way. In everyday life, in the absence of theoretical or explanatory models, guilt is normally associated with a highly personal, penance-based response to previous mis*deeds* (hence its typical association with morality and with a sense of self-imposed correctness or autonomy). Bernard Williams, in his roundabout characterization of the emotion – and also because he has Kant and Kantian philosophers as specific targets of his analysis – links its manifestation at the personal level to an immediate acknowledgement of breaches of the moral law. Contrary to what we find in his broad account of shame and its moral relevance, his understanding of guilt is tied to an acknowledgement of moral principles, and he builds his analysis within a framework of morality qua system of normative principles and rules. At no point in his strategic depiction of the experience of guilt does Williams make room for what one might call an 'attack of guilt' (just as it is common to speak of 'panic attacks'), which is closer to the kind of guilt experience portrayed by Dodds.

With the analysis of this *mental* and *moral* experience from the first section in hand, it is clear both that we – moral agents well into the twenty-first century, with a whole range of unprecedented worries and fears – can make sense of the experience ascribed to the Archaic Greeks in *The Greeks and the Irrational* and that we can recognize both its occurrence in and its relevance to our shared moral stories.

The problem with Bernard Williams's marginal analysis of guilt and guilt responses within *Shame and Necessity* lies perhaps in the fact that he does with this emotion what he accuses Kantian moral philosophers – or classical scholars with an unbending bias towards Kantianism in moral matters – of doing with the ethical frameworks developed in ancient philosophy, poetry and drama: He takes a moralized definition of guilt for granted, leaving aside the more nuanced aspects of the emotion that some classical scholars before him took seriously.

Paying close attention to Williams's own words, one can see where the roots of the problem with his definition of the mechanisms of guilt lie. On page 223 of *Shame and Necessity* – quoted above – we read the following statement:

> When the conception of guilt is refined beyond a certain point and *forgets its primitive materials of anger and fear*, guilt comes to be represented simply as the attitude of respect for an abstract law, and it then no longer has any special connection with victims.[16]

To the extent that Williams chooses to depict guilt as an abstract response to violations of the moral law, he leaves out of consideration the very real possibility that guilt may be a rich, ethically responsible type of emotional feedback to wrongs done to (concrete) others – one that preserves the 'primitive materials of anger and fear' while keeping the victims of our past misdeeds consistently in sight.

On all counts, it is the somewhat narrow Kantian and moralized inflection of his indirect analysis of guilt – in addition to the fact that shame is his primary focus – that prevents Williams from considering different kinds of first-personal experiences of the emotion, including straightforward responses to specific cases of wrongdoing and an attitude of penance towards particular victims. Due to the classical background that informs his reading of different types of irrational experience in the Greek worldview, Dodds himself is not directly interested in the role played by victims in his preferred account of guilt-feelings. He leaves the door open to their inclusion, however. The simple presence of psychoanalytical material in his analysis of the irrationality of guilt and his theoretical borrowing of Freudian ideas keeps Dodds's analytical framework within the bounds of personal and psychological ideas about the emotion.[17] Whether for cosmological and deeply religious reasons (as with the stories of well-known characters from Greek tragedies and myths) or for secular psychological reasons (prevailing in contemporary societies), his acute description of the *maddening* features that underlie experiences of guilt preserves the structural interpersonal strata of direct relations between man and the gods, or between man and man. (Of course, when he borrows from psychoanalytical sources, Dodds has in mind family relations and their relevance to one's mental and moral life.)[18]

Williams's effort to secularize an account of moral emotions (even if borrowing from classical mythological and religious material) while criticizing Kantian analytical sources prevents him from appreciating the richness of alternative phenomenologies of both shame and guilt in the classical scholarship that inspired him. Dodds is a case in point in this respect – although surely not the only one.[19] His keen insistence that guilt-feelings may be a direct response to personal instances of *hybris* or unwarranted (or excessive) self-assertion, leading to voluntary punishment and the mending of one's ways – if need be by a set of cathartic or self-purifying measures – is both a rich alternative conception of guilt and thoroughly familiar to the contemporary moral agent. It adds up to a view according to which the central role of the victims of one's misdeeds is consistently preserved. Making amends when my moral misbehavior has affected *someone* keeps the figure of my moral interlocutor in sight (perhaps focusing my attention on him/her in undistorted and non-generalizable ways).

Finally, two elements that have been left out of consideration thus far must still be accounted for. One is the personal impact that the experience of guilt described by Dodds can have on one's ethical (and moral) behavior, especially in avoiding the dramatic consequences that its absence could entail; the other is an accommodation of this kind of guilt experience in the structural layout of Williams's criticism of the 'Morality System'.[20]

At the outset of this chapter, I referred to the danger of the moral and mental self-destruction to which unresolved feelings of guilt can lead. It is indeed a virtue of Dodds's unconventional analysis of guilt and guilt-mechanisms that it highlights the rehabilitative power that psychologically binding responses to disturbing feelings of guilt can have when it comes to one's ethical and even moral – that is, duty-bound – behavior. When concentrating on key aspects of the moral psychology of characters in Greek classical tragedy and transposing the structural mechanism of guilt-responses found therein to a modern moral protagonist and to a modern moral outlook, Dodds registers the potential for moral self-destruction that inheres in irrational, but psychologically determining, feelings of guilt. This notion figures prominently in the above quotation from *Antigone*, and its inspiration and modern follow-up, borrowed from a Freudian psychoanalytic framework,[21] lends it both prominence and a sound theoretical background. Although Dodds's analysis does not explicitly refer to the specifically *healing* (or self-correcting) power of guilt in guilt-cultures (partly because he ends this lecture in a highly speculative tone), a reading of his model informed by therapeutic aims is not unimaginable. And if the dangers of maddening or overwhelming episodes of guilt are stressed in his own account of instances of the emotion, the notion that these risks can be avoided by respecting its moral precepts is equally inferable from everything Dodds chooses to say about primitive responses to deep psychological pressures. Avoiding or overcoming guilt and its collateral damage to the individual psyche may lead to moral and mental well-being, on the positive side of moral commitments and individual responses to particular situations (a feat that would be welcomed by an anti-moralist like Bernard Williams).

The determining presence of guilt within guilt-cultures, the psychologically normative layout of which is introduced by Dodds's pioneering study, adds a level of nuance to feelings of guilt that is absent in Bernard Williams's impoverished remarks on the emotion. By choosing to focus on (and attack) a moralized account of guilt in Kantian terms, Williams misses the opportunity – which he rightly pursues with regard to shame – to imaginatively elaborate richer phenomenological descriptions of the emotion and to consider how they might benefit the ethical life of the agent (and even of *victims*), an insight that we find in Dodds's analysis. Marginalized as a key but highly damaging outcome of the Morality System[22] and its unbending focus on the idea of moral obligation, guilt is, in Williams's framework, portrayed as an emotional pattern we would do well to be rid of (or, at the very least, to prevent from dominating us). In the strict terms of his analysis, this conclusion is not unwarranted. When our frame of reference is widened to cover certain analytic details of other sources from twentieth-century scholarship – including sources unblemished by Williams's account and criticism – his model is suddenly revealed as insufficiently critical and even historically unfair to some of his predecessors and sources of inspiration. Eric Dodds is a case in point in this regard.

Concluding remarks

This chapter has presented (and expanded upon) alternative descriptions and interpretations of the moral and psychological value of feelings of *guilt* as described by two preeminent twentieth-century scholars of ancient thought – especially ancient moral thought: Eric Dodds and Bernard Williams. I have suggested that both of their readings of this moral emotion are insufficient in their own terms. Furthermore, given what both thinkers have to say about guilt and guilt-feelings, it is clear that simply complementing one model with the other will not on its own provide us with a proper or richer view of the emotion. Although teacher and pupil, Dodds and Williams put forth very different conceptions of what is involved in the experience of guilt – at least in the two texts I have chosen to bring together in the present analysis.

One element that is crucial to Dodds's model, as we have seen, is the extent to which guilt can either lead to or arise out of insanity and even be a sign of personal madness beyond repair. *The Greeks and the Irrational*, in line with other anthropological masterpieces written about the same time, depicts features of classical Greek society and gives details of the Greek mentality and moral psychology in terms that contrast deeply with our contemporary moral outlook – including emotional patterns that we recognize as belonging to our ethical lives.

In Dodds's study, guilt is presented as an emotional background that can span generations and damage the reputations of heroes – although its structural features are traceable to emotional reactions we sometimes have or can come to have when something minor goes wrong with one's ethical reactions. Through careful comparison, this chapter has shown that a defining structure of the ancient moral paradigm is easily recovered and recognized in our shared secular moral experiences, in those cases where a delicate emotional balance has not been reached (or where a balanced framework has been disturbed). In other words: episodes of deep personal guilt may make the subject prey to mental imbalances that, in terms of gravity, are akin to those that afflict the Sophoclean hero. Nevertheless, due to its mental force and dominance, guilt may equally serve as a rescue of sorts in terms of relocating one's (arguably) lost moral thread. In this sense, although neglected by some, guilt may in fact be an indispensable moral incentive.[23]

Finally – as argued above – when it assumes such pressing phenomenological contours, the sort of abstract dangers that were pointed out in Bernard Williams's indirect Kantian analysis of guilt as a moral emotion all fall away. Guilt is now not an abstract deference to the moral law but an impetus to mend one's moral ways. As such, it is an emotional response with both moral content and, precisely because of this, moral value.

Notes

1 The distinction between 'shame-cultures' and 'guilt-cultures' was first spoken of by Ruth Benedict in *The Chrysanthemum and the Sword* (Benedict, 1946) and is described at great length by Eric Dodds in the second lecture of *The Greeks and the Irrational.*

2 Solon (Greek: Σόλων; 638 BCE–558 BCE) was an Athenian statesman, lawmaker and poet. He is best known for his efforts to legislate against political, economic and moral decline in Archaic Athens. His reforms failed in the short term, but he is often credited with having laid the foundations for Athenian democracy in the sixth century BCE.

3 Bernard Williams gave the Sather Lectures at Berkeley in 1989, published in 1993 as *Shame and Necessity*. In these lectures, he argued for a thoughtful reconsideration of shame as a fundamental moral response in both the classical and the modern moral outlook, against the kind of Judeo-Christian moral framework, which tends to put guilt at the core of morality. Arguing against contemporary attacks on ancient ethical outlooks, Williams offers a very unfavorable notion of guilt, viewed as unhealthy self-punishment.

4 In the *Diagnostic and Statistical Manual of Mental Disorders* (DSM-5), 'Delirium' is defined as 'a neurocognitive disorder that opens a mental crisis with different possible etiological causes and subtypes' (DSM, 93).

5 In a famous essay from 1977, Anthony O'Hear defines guilt as follows: 'A man is said to be guilty when he has broken some law or code by which he is bound, as a result of which he incurs a liability to punishment. Guilt itself is like a burden or a pollution which can be removed only by undergoing the appropriate punishment or by being forgiven by the appropriate authority' (O'Hear, 1977, 73).

6 For a recent set of models to account for the cluster idea of 'moral shock', see *The Politics of Emotional Shockwaves*, esp. chs. 8 and 9 (Falcato & Graça da Silva, 2021).

7 Soph. *Ant.* 583ff.

8 Schematically, and in arguing for the moral relevance of shame while unearthing the deep structures of shame-feelings and shame-behavior, Williams's study offers a kind of Nietzschean deconstructive model of modern moral outlooks – one that involves the reassessment of pre-Socratic philosophical ideas and that attacks a system the core emotional foundation of which is guilt as unnecessarily castrating and damaging to the moral agent.

9 See esp. Arthur Adkins, 1960, 1970.

10 See Williams, 1993: 75–102.

11 See Williams, 2011: 60–79.

12 Italics mine.

13 On his approach to guilt and in all he has to say about shame and its impact on personal moral conduct, Bernard Williams never explicitly draws on (let alone quotes) texts written by Kant himself, specifically those texts in which Kant directly comments on both shame and guilt (see Falcato, 2021).

14 See Williams, 1993, 93–94: 'If we come to understand our shame, we may also better understand our guilt. The structures of shame contain the possibility of controlling and learning from guilt, because they give a conception of one's ethical identity, in relation to which guilt can make sense. Shame can understand guilt, but guilt cannot understand itself. ... *To the modern moral consciousness*, guilt seems a more transparent moral emotion than shame. It may

seem so, but that is only because, as it presents itself, it is more isolated than shame is from other elements of one's self-image, the rest of one's desires and needs, and because it leaves out a lot even of one's ethical consciousness. It can direct one towards those who have been wronged or damaged, and demand reparation in the name, simply, of what has happened to them. But it cannot by itself help one to understand one's relations to those happenings, or to rebuild the self that has done these things and the world in which that self has to live. Only shame can do that, because it embodies conceptions of what one is and of how one is related to others.'

15 Bernard Williams's work on ethics *and* moral philosophy – he insisted on keeping the two notions and their specific sources of normativity apart – is known for having revived ancient ways of thinking about the 'good life' and for downplaying the narrowness of modern approaches to morality – just as Dodds does in his study (see Williams, 2011, ch. 10; Williams, 1993).

16 Williams, 1993: 223, italics mine.

17 See Dodds, 1951: 45–50.

18 See Dodds, 1951: 47–48: 'For, to begin with, the human father had from the earliest times his heavenly counterpart: Zeus *pater* belongs to the Indo-European inheritance, as his Latin and Sanskrit equivalents indicate; and Calhoun has shown how closely the status and conduct of the Homeric Zeus is modelled on that of the Homeric paterfamilias. ... It was natural to project on to the heavenly Father those curious mixed feelings about the human one which the child dared not acknowledge even to himself'.

19 Considering only the great historical systematizers of ethics or moral philosophy, both Aristotle and Kant have more ideas about both emotional patterns than Williams gives them credit for (see Kant, 2007; Aristotle, 2011).

20 This, we have seen, is systematically presented in the last chapter of *Ethics and the Limits of Philosophy* and is dismissively labeled as the 'Peculiar Institution', although hints of it are equally present in the analysis of features of Greek ethical life highlighted in *Shame and Necessity*.

21 See Dodds, 1951, 47–49: 'You see perhaps where all this is tending. The psychologists have taught us how potent a source of guilt-feelings is the pressure of unacknowledged desires, desires which are excluded from consciousness save in dreams or daydreams, yet are able to produce in the self a deep sense of moral uneasiness. This uneasiness often takes a religious form today; and if a similar feeling existed in Archaic Greece, this would be the natural form for it to take. ... In the meantime, I shall not complain if classical scholars shake their heads over the foregoing remarks. And, to avoid misunderstanding, I would in conclusion emphasize two things. First, I do not expect this particular key, or any key, to open all doors. The evolution of a culture is too complex a thing to be explained without residue in terms of any simple formula, whether economic or psychological, begotten of Marx or begotten of Freud. We must resist the temptation to simplify what is not simple. And secondly, to explain origins is not to explain away values. We should beware of underrating the religious significance of the ideas I have discussed to-day, even where, like the doctrine of divine temptation, they are repugnant to our moral sense.'

22 See Williams, 2011: 193ff.

23 See its notorious absence from a recent issue on the topic of neglected moral emotions (Elpidorou, 2020).

Bibliography

Adkins, A. H. (1960). *Merit and Responsibility: A Study in Greek Values*. Oxford: Clarendon Press.

——— (1970). *From the Many to the One: A Study of Personality and Views of Human Nature in the Context of Ancient Greek Society*. New York: Cornell University Press.

Aristotle (2011). *Nichomachean Ethics*. Trans. Robert C. Bartlett and Susan Collins. Chicago and London: The University of Chicago Press.

Benedict, Ruth (1946; 2005). *The Chrysanthemum and the Sword: Patterns of Japanese Culture*. New York: Mariner Books, 2005.

Beck, Lewis W. (1960). *A Commentary on Kant's Critique of Practical Reason*. Chicago and London: The University of Chicago Press.

Cavell, Stanley (1976). *Must we Mean What We Say? A Book of Essays*. Cambridge: Cambridge University Press.

Dodds, Eric (1951). *The Greeks and the Irrational*. Berkeley and Los Angeles: University of California Press.

——— (1977). *Missing Persons: An Autobiography*. Oxford: Clarendon Press.

Elpidorou, Andreas (2020). 'Neglected Emotions'. *The Monist*, 103(2), 135–146. https://doi.org/10.1093/monist/onz031

Euripides (2007). *Alcestis, Medea, Hippolytus*. Trans. Diane Arnson Svarlien. Indianapolis: Hackett Publishing Co.

Falcato, Ana Cristina (2021). 'Die Idee des Schaminstinkts in Kants anthropologischen Schriften'. *Deutsche Zeitschrift für Philosophie*, 69(3), 383–402. https://doi.org/10.1515/dzph-2021-0032

Falcato, A. & Graça da Silva, S. (Eds.) (2021). *The Politics of Emotional Shockwaves*. London: Palgrave Macmillan. https://doi.org/10.1007/978-3-030-56021-8

Kant, Immanuel (2015). *Critique of Practical Reason*. Trans. Mary Gregor; introduction by Andrews Reath. Cambridge: Cambridge University Press.

——— (2002). *Groundwork for the Metaphysics of Morals*. Ed. Thomas E. Hill, Jr. and Arnulf Zweig. Oxford: Oxford University Press.

——— (2007). 'Anthropology, History, and Education'. In *The Cambridge Edition of the Works of Immanuel Kant*. Ed. Günter Zöller and Robert B. Louden. Cambridge: Cambridge University Press.

——— (2003). *Religion Within the Boundaries of Mere Reason: And Other Writings*. Trans. and Ed. Allen Wood and George di Giovanni. Cambridge: Cambridge University Press.

Lear, Jonathan (2006). 'Psychoanalysis and the Idea of a Moral Psychology: Memorial to Bernard Williams' Philosophy'. *Inquiry*, 47, 515–522.

O'Brien, L. (2020). 'Shameful self-consciousness'. *European Journal of Philosophy*, 28, 545–566.

O'Hear, Anthony (1977). 'Guilt and Shame as Moral Concepts'. *Proceedings of the Aristotelian Society*, 77, 73–86.

Sartre, Jean-Paul (1992). *Being and Nothingness*. New York: Washington Square Press.

Scheler, Max (1957). 'Über Scham und Schamgefühl'. In *Schriften aus dem Nachlass, vol. I: Zur Ethik und Erkenntnislehre*. Bern: Francke Verlag.

Szigeti, Andras & Talbert, Matthew (Eds.). (2022). *Morality and Agency: Themes from Bernard Williams*. Oxford: OUP.

Williams, Bernard (1993). *Shame and Necessity*. Berkeley, CA: University of California Press.

——— (2011). *Ethics and the Limits of Philosophy*. London and New York: Routledge Classics.

——— (1973). *Problems of the Self: Philosophical Papers 1956–1972*. Cambridge: Cambridge University Press.

——— (1957). 'Morality and the Emotions'. In *Problems of the Self: Philosophical Papers 1956–1972*. Cambridge: Cambridge University Press.

4 Ancient, Medieval and Early Modern Ideas about Delusional Thought in Burton's *Anatomy*

Jennifer Radden

Introduction

Robert Burton was an English clergyman and scholar living in the beginning of the seventeenth century.[1] His life work – the great *Anatomy of Melancholy* – aimed to preserve ancient, medieval and renaissance medical knowledge and lore about the disordered states of mind, mood and behavior known as Melancholy. The *Anatomy* is much else besides, including a self-help health guide and a literary satire. But in my own work on Burton from which the following chapter has been excerpted, attention is to his close explication of classic writing about delusional states. Hippocratic aphorisms, Aristotelian faculty psychology about the imagination, the medieval Arab thinker Avicenna and later renaissance doctors such as Du Laurens are all brought to bear as Burton tries to encapsulate past understanding of the puzzling symptoms associated with delusional thought. These ideas, and some of their obvious links to theorizing about delusions within today's mind sciences of philosophy, psychiatry and cognitive psychology are the subject of what follows.

Delusions still elude medical science; even today, we are short of agreed-upon and comprehensive explanatory models or reliable and effective treatment. Arguably then, we cannot afford to disregard the analyses and ideas assiduously gathered by Burton from the eras pre-dating modern medical science. While providing no reliable epidemiological evidence from his era, Burton's enquiry serves, I will show, to illuminate questions about the structure and antecedents of delusional thought over which there is still considerable debate.

Central themes within Burton's many references to delusional thinking are introduced in Part 1. In Part 2 these are discussed in relation to some present-day research, followed by a brief note on delusions and dreams.

DOI: 10.4324/9781003288992-6

Part 1

"When Reason also is corrupted"

The *Anatomy* is filled with, and enlivened by, tales of those who have fallen prey to misapprehensions of delusional proportions: the woman said to have thought she swallowed a serpent, the gentleman who was "afraid to pisse, least all the towne should be drowned," the man who supposed his nose so big that he should "dash it against the wall if he stirred" and one who believed he was dead (II,2,6,3:112). In this chapter we'll look at what Burton says about these extreme states of disorder. If reason cannot be exerted the way it should, he explains, then in cases like these, not merely imagination but reason itself has become corrupted.

Careless and self-indulgent uses of the imagination place anyone at risk of succumbing to habitual Melancholy; we are all in that respect potentially *akratic* melancholics. But Burton loosely separates the less advanced states and tendencies we have within our power to avert and control, from the habituated, chronic condition that is the subject of the present chapter. Melancholic men, Burton says, see and hear so many phantasms, chimeras, noises, and visions, that

> their corrupt fantasy makes them see and hear that which indeed is neither heard nor seen.
>
> (I,3,3, 1:424)

This is melancholy the habit, which is beyond self-help. Our judgment has become "so depraved, our reason over-ruled, Will precipitated, that we *cannot seeke our owne good, or moderate our selves*" (II,2,6,1:104, emphasis added). Indeed, it may be beyond any help:

> you may as well bid him that is diseased not to feel pain, as a melancholy man not to fear, not to be sad: 'tis within his blood, his brains, his whole temperature, it *cannot be removed.*
>
> (II,2,6,1: 103)

Burton mostly suggests that cases of delusional and hallucinatory experience involve melancholy, rather than outright madness. Although many writers "make *Madnesse* and *Melancholy* but one Disease," he explains, he will follow the newer thinkers ("our neotericks") who handle them apart" (I,1,4:132). In light of this resolve, the passage asserting that some melancholic men "are mad" is best understood to imply that severe cases of melancholy can become madness, which he readily admits elsewhere.[2]

Where these states would be assigned according to today's disorder categories is also a matter of potential confusion. In the *Anatomy*, Melancholy is distinguished from madness in terms of its predominant moods of sadness and fear and its relative lack of vehemence and violence. Today, by contrast, more severe states of disorder are most often distinguished clinically by the presence of psychotic features (along with indications of social and behavioral dysfunction), identified through evidence of delusions and hallucinations. And although they occur in psychotic depression, delusions and hallucinations are less commonly associated with mood disorder than with schizophrenia and related conditions, categories not in use until after the early modern period. Burton's admission that some melancholic men might be mad seems to better fit this later rubric (where, indeed, psychosis is aligned in common parlance with the less polite "madness"). However, historians assure us that in seventeenth-century England, these delusional states would not have been judged as mad.[3] Madness might be the eventual outcome of severe Melancholy. But as defined in the *Anatomy*, madness had a violence and vehemence not present, even in cases of severe melancholy.

Retrospective diagnosis holds many dangers, fostered by the lure of the "continuity mirage" involving the common (but groundless) "belief that irrespective of historical period terms such as ... *melancholia* ... *hysteria*, or *fatigue* must refer to more or less the same 'clinical' phenomena" (Berrios 2011:xv).[4]

To avoid those dangers, it is sufficient to conclude here that many of Burton's tales depict symptoms delusional enough that they would be classed as indicative of severe disorder today.

Melancholy in Habit

The all-encompassing and flexible humoral system allows Burton to identify as Melancholy states of disorder according to four different dimensions. They are more and less permanent, more and less severe and dysfunctional, more and less intractable, and more and less temperamentally engendered. This is useful for his account, but it invites confusion. At the beginning of the *Anatomy*, he takes some care with distinctions:

> Melancholy ... is either in Disposition, or Habit. In Disposition, is that transitory Melancholy, which goes & comes upon every small occasion of sorrow, need, sickness, trouble, fear, grief, passion, or perturbation of the Mind ... from these Melancholy Dispositions, no man living is free. ... This Melancholy of which we are to treat, as in Habit ... a Chronic or continuate disease, a settled humor ... not errant but fixed, and as it was long increasing, so now being (pleasant, or painful) grown to an habit, it will hardly be removed.

While acknowledging that the one can lead to the other, Burton here promises that his work will be limited to melancholy properly so called, that is, understood as disease (Melancholy the Habit). He falls short in this resolve, and the book is unwieldy, but more interesting and valuable, as a result. As is implied in much of the *Anatomy*, however, melancholy properly so called (the habit) is, in some sense, disease and aberration, in contrast to the many normal passing states that, while resembling it, result from life's vicissitudes. (Even these may be quite slight when combined with an inherently melancholy temperament.) Several pairs of contrasts thus occur in this dense passage, corresponding to the dimensions noted above. The general contrast between states that are passing and those that are more chronic is the broadest one, with application to both normal and abnormal states. A normal, passing or "errant" state may grow into a habit, as he puts it. Through our own doing, when we indulge "melancholizing" tendencies and allow them to go unchecked, it might become an abnormal, intractable condition. Other times, and similar states in other people, will be passing and insignificant in their effects, never becoming chronic diseases in this sense. In addition, both passing and longer-term feelings of melancholy may reflect nothing more than normal responses to the inevitable occasions of, as he says, sorrow, need, sickness, trouble, fear, grief, passion or perturbation of the mind.

In addition, there are those with inherited melancholy temperament ("borne of Melancholy parents" [I,1,2,3:165]). Reviewing ancient medical authorities on the contribution of parents as the cause of melancholy, Burton concludes: "I need not therefore make any doubt of Melancholy, but that it is an hereditary disease" (I,2,1,6:206). The melancholy temperament of the seventeenth century – described as sober, contemplative, and timorous – was thought to stem from an abundance of the "natural" form of the melancholy humor, rather than its corrupted, "adust" form.[5] In addition to the temperament we receive from our parents (at I,2,1,6: 205), Burton acknowledges a host of the causes of Melancholy that we are powerless to avoid, those from angels, devils, the alignment of the stars, God, and witches, as well as old age. Added to these, and just as multitudinous, are causes we can avoid through the practice of healthy daily habits.

Like the separation between habit and disposition, the division between temperament and more occasional states can be expressed without reference to humoral language, and exhibits obvious parallels with today's language of genetic and other endogenous risk factors for disorders such as depression. There is a difference, though, in that the four humoral temperaments were not in themselves abnormalities. By contrast, even the dysthymic temperament is often regarded as pathology within medical psychiatry today. (Peter Kramer, for example, insists that because the number, severity, and duration of depressive episodes "sit on a continuum of risk" they all form, as he says, part of "a single picture," and we ought to understand their manifestations "*as pathology all along the spectrum*" [2005: 166, 170]. Kramer's reasoning here is based on research showing that early depression is, as he says, both a disease and a risk factor: a predictor of future, and worsening episodes.[6]) Illustrating such reasoning, the trait-based disposition towards pessimism and sadness, formerly known as Dysthymia, has been merged with Chronic Major Disorder in the most recent psychiatric classification (DSM-5). This yielded the composite Persistent Depressive Disorder: a chronic form of depression whose diagnostic feature is "depressed mood for most of the day, for more days than not," for at least two years in adults, and one in children. (APA 2013:168).

The passage where Burton lays out these different ways Melancholy is to be understood, goes on to explain that the term "melancholy" has looser and more precise uses:

> In which *Equivocal and improper* sense, we call him Melancholy, that is dull, sad, sowre, lumpish, ill disposed, solitary, any way moved, or displeased. ... Melancholy in this sense is the Character of Mortalitie.
> (italics added)

Only in its loose, equivocal, and improper sense is Melancholy an inescapable aspect of human experience.

Delusional States of Fear and Sadness

As used by Burton, "Melancholy" was an expansive category extending beyond the mood disorders of present-day psychiatric classifications. Nonetheless, affective states, particularly those of sadness and fear without cause, had been associated with the black bile since Hippocratic times. While not exclusive to it, disordered moods lie at the center of Burton's analysis because of the relation they bear to the imagination and reason in his Aristotelian faculty psychology.

Moods of nebulous, seemingly objectless apprehension known as free-floating anxiety are familiar today, yet they are barely recognizable among Burton's examples. Cases of fear in the *Anatomy* have precise, although usually fanciful, objects. Today, we would count them delusional or the creatures of delusional thought processes. Their themes run along familiar lines: guilt, impending disasters stemming from personal attributes or unavoidable circumstances, as well as excessive responses, mountains made of molehills – misapprehensions that provide reasons, albeit bad ones, for the states of distress that accompany them. These are fears "without cause." They are without sufficient cause, in excess of, or inappropriate to, their cause.

Burton was a story-teller, and little of importance about the symptom picture of melancholy, let alone about seventeenth-century epidemiology, can probably be drawn from these examples.[7] In particular, they cannot reliably guide us as to the frequency of delusion-based fears and worries in contrast to the presence of dejection and sadness – or (the more literal interpretation of "without cause") to the prevalence of nebulous moods without any apparent or recognizable object. The strange and wonderful fears that resulted from bizarre delusional beliefs make for more lively reading than accounts of the mopish moods of downhearted melancholics. Viewed as epidemiological data, the apparent prevalence of single-themed or delusions observed by some commentators seems likely to be similarly wanting. Citing the man who supposes himself made of butter and fears he will melt in the sun;[8] the one frightened that he will "speake aloud ... something indecent" during a sermon,[9] or he who fears he is suspected of imaginary crimes,[10] Christopher Tilmouth concludes that a single obsession "dogs the imagination" (Tilmouth 2005:529). Certainly, the habit of "melancholizing" frequently described by Burton will ensure that these distorted ideas are dwelt on repetitively. Moreover, some habitual melancholy is in one passage described as having lucid intervals (II:3,8,1: 206). And in another, Burton describes some sufferers who, although otherwise of "impregnable wits ... and discreet," in their particular idea or obsession, "[the] madnesse and folly breakes out beyond measure" (III,4,1,3:388). But again, we are not told enough to assess the extent of the delusional thought patterns that might have been associated with these cases. And whether, for example, they more closely correspond to what are today often distinguished as limited *monothematic* delusions, or more elaborated *polythematic* ones remains unclear.[11]

When delusions have become entrenched (our judgment depraved, as Burton says, our reason over-ruled), and self-control is temporarily lost ("the Will precipitated"), efforts at self-help must prove fruitless. His cases include milder melancholic states as well, but Burton frequently describes obsessions and bizarre ideas that would today be deemed evidence of psychosis. And he joins other thinkers from before and since his time in identifying a disordered imagination, not merely – and apparently not always – disordered reason, as the source of the aberrant thinking we associate with delusion. In all melancholy men, Burton says, referring to their natural temperament, the faculty of imagination is "most Powerful and strong." But in melancholy as disease, it is excessively so, producing "strange conceptions and absurd shapes." The misapprehensions that arise this way are bizarre and extreme, about people who

> suppose they have no heads, flye, sinke, they are pots, glasses, &c. is wind in their heads."
>
> (I,3,3,1:420)

The imagination produces not only these delusional ideas, but sensory-based hallucinations as well. Some melancholy men

> have a corrupt eare – they think they hear musicke, or some hideous noise as their phantasie conceaves, corrupt eyes, some smelling: some one sense, some another. *Lewis* the Eleventh had a conceat everything did stinke about him; all the odiferous perfumes they could get would not ease him, but still he smelled a filthy stinke.
>
> (I,3,1,3:402)

An over-active imagination explains all melancholy tendencies, even milder ones, however. And it is equally the source of valuable forms of creativity and self-healing. So how is this point to be identified at which all self-control is lost? Burton gives two kinds of answer to that question. One resorts to the criterion of self-care or self-governance. Those with such extreme misapprehensions are (at least temporarily) beyond helping themselves, and must turn to others. A second, seemingly more precise account, suggests that the point of separation involves the parts played by imagination and reason, respectively. Once reason has become corrupted, then the creations of the imagination cannot be corrected – by ourselves or our friends. Arguably, these two approaches reflect degrees of disease severity. When the imagination alone is disturbed, friends can sometimes help, as we'll see below. But when reason is itself corrupted, even friends will be powerless.

The role of friends in averting and expunging the apprehensions of the melancholic, carefully explained in the *Anatomy*, takes us some way in understanding the kind of entrenched and habituated melancholy that is beyond any help we can undertake *on our own*, cases where "the heart will not lay aside these vicious motions, and the phantasy those fond imaginings." In that circumstance, we have "another form of government to enforce and refrain our outward members, that they be not led by our passions." At such times,

> our judgement be so depraved, our reason overruled, will precipitated, that we cannot *seek our own good*, or moderate ourselves. ... [T]he best way for ease is to impart our misery to some friend, not smother it up in our own breast ... for grief concealed strangles the soul; but whereas we shall but import it to some discreet, trusty, loving friend, it is instantly removed, by his counsel haply, wisdom, persuasion, advice, his good means, which we could not otherwise apply unto ourselves.
>
> (II, 2,6,2 emphasis added)

The effects of friendship on the imagination explain how this works,

> Friends confabulations are comfortable at all times. ... [T]he simplest narration many times easeth our distressed mind, and ... *a faithful friend ... sees that which we cannot see for passion and discontent*, he pacifies our minds, he will ease our pain, assuage our anger.
>
> (II,2,6,2, emphasis added)

The friend offers us a clearer view, he (or she) sees what we are temporarily blinded to: feelings of friendship embody expectations and attitudes that are hopeful and reassuring. Only when the person is not able to resist or overcome these heart-eating passions, Burton goes on, "his friends *or physician* must be ready to supply that which is wanting" (emphasis added). Although physicians are included, what follows makes it clear that Burton supposes friends of equal or greater value here. He quotes Hippocrates: physicians alone cannot effect a cure ("They must all joyne") and explains that a melancholy discontented person must

> not bee left unto themselves, but with some company or other, least by that meanes they aggravate and increase their disease.
>
> (II,2,6,2:106)

The more obvious duties of friendship in such a situation are enumerated: friends and companions must be especially aware of the discontented person, not leave him with strangers, alone or idle, divert his thoughts with " some businesse, exercise or recreation." (II, 2,6,2: 107). More precise recommendations then follow: these deal with the distorted beliefs and misapprehensions that come with severe melancholy when the sufferer's weakness "be such that he cannot discern what is amiss, correct, or satisfy." In that circumstance, it behooves friends,

> by counsell, comfort, or perswasion, by faire or foule meanes, to alienate his minde, by some artificiall invention, or some contrary perswasion, to remove all objects, causes, companies, occasions, as may any waies molest him, to humour him, please him, divert him, and if it be possible, by altering his course of life, to give him security and satisfaction.
>
> (II, 2,6,2:107)

The obligations of friends can thus be quite considerable, even burdensome. They will take time, and attentive, thoughtful effort. They may also be disagreeable, testing the friendship in other ways, the reference to "fair means or foul," indicates. Burton countenanced the deceptions commonly employed in his times, as we saw earlier. "Sometimes ... by some feigned lie, strange news, witty device, artificial invention, it is not amiss to deceive them," he expands (II,2,6,2:111). Approvingly, he offers examples: there was the woman who thought she had swallowed a serpent, was made to vomit, and given to believe that she succeeded in expelling the creature, after which she was cured. In our later, more modern times, respect for the patient's dignity prevents such subterfuge, and these deceitful practices on the part of anyone would be unacceptable. Apparently ready to ignore the dubious aspect of the practice in such dire circumstances, Burton applauds it as a demonstration of the power of imagination and suggestion. With this and several other examples, he is unabashedly intent to show such deceptions work.[12] But this not only elevates friendship well beyond where we would today assign it. It also seems to show a pre-modern disregard for the demands of what we would today recognize as the moral integrity of the friend, and the dignity of the melancholic sufferer.

When self-care fails ("we cannot seek our owne good, moderate our selves"), there are always friends, then. And friends play a number of roles, not all of which we would endorse for the treatment of any disorder today. Beyond that, some disorder, when it is "within his blood, his brains, his whole temperature" may be without remedy. Then, it "cannot be removed."

Two-Factor Analyses: "Imagination or reason, alone, or both"[13]

There is also a more technical answer to the question of when severe, and likely incurable disorder, sets in. That the imagination is somehow deficient is not doubted. Because such extreme imaginings would usually be kept in check by reason, however, not merely a runaway imagination but a failure or lapse of reason must be invoked for a complete explanation of these errors, Burton explains. Learned debates over whether delusion ("the affection") "be imagination or reason alone, or both," are reviewed. Galen's view is that melancholy primarily affects the imagination, while others are named as believing that the understanding is the damaged faculty. In his words,

> reason was in fault as well as Imagination, which did not correct this error. ... Why doth not reason detect the fallacy, settle and persuade, if she be free? Avicenna therefore holds both corrupt, to whom most Arabians subscribe ... no man doubts of Imagination, but that it is hurt and misaffected here.
>
> (1,1,3,2: 164-5)

Appealing to the authority of Avicenna and the other scholars in his tradition, Burton here postulates that reason, on particular occasions, has lost control of the melancholic's wild imaginings.[14] Here, reason itself is somehow more deeply compromised, so it not only fails to, but *cannot*, engage in its usual function of curbing and correcting. The exact deficiencies attributed to reason and the imagination in these passages are not entirely clear. And Burton's elaboration about those occasions when the humor has become heated or *adusted* do not substantially advance our understanding, although the smoky vapors that distort our reasoning with adustion are equally beyond the correction we might expect from Reason. Quoting from renaissance thinker Thomas Wright (1986), he explains that the mind is in these cases confined "within a perpetuall dungeon," and oppressed with "continuall feares, anxieties, sorrowes, &c." (I,3,3,1:419) because it has become entrenched. Such melancholy men have not true object of feare, but an "inward cause" within them (I,3,3,1:420).

Even today, delusional thinking lacks a clear-cut and agreed-upon definition, and is incompletely understood.[15] However, present-day mind science regularly identifies several parts that go wrong in sustained delusions. A collection of problems attach to the initial, delusional idea involving its often implausible content, and the means of its acquisition, in ungrounded flashes of intuition, as well as by evidently implausible reasoning. Then there is the unaccountable tenacity with which the notion often continues to be embraced despite the disconfirming evidence provided by the epistemic community, common sense, or past experience.[16]

This second defect allows delusions to become entrenched beliefs, or belief-like (the matter of how to describe them is contested), rather than being dismissed as passing fancies and illusions. It is a failure to "detect the fallacy, settle and persuade," as Burton puts it. That the implausibility and tenacity exhibited when there is sustained delusional thought somehow correspond to these separate functions of imagining and reasoning identified by Burton seems beyond doubt. The imagination is responsible for conjuring up the original, strange ideas, whereas the process by which they are maintained in the face of countervailing evidence reflects a malfunction of reasoning. Reason, as Burton says, should have corrected the error. Alone, the products of the imagination are innocuous. It is by assenting and blindly clinging to them that we fall into states of error that indicate disease. So Burton's account differs little from contemporary analyses in these broad categories.

What is also clear here is that the separated failures of reasoning and imagining are *initiated* by a flawed imagination. About the causal relation between and direction of their respective deficiencies, Burton quotes "a learned doctor of Padua," concluding that if the disease be chronic (" inveterate, or ... more or less of continuance "),

> "I determine ... that it is first in Imagination, and afterwards in reason."

Any later effects, including those on reason, are thus secondary ("accidental"). Appealing to another authority (Herc. De Saxonia), Burton concludes that the imagination is the source of all the errors that follow:

> Faith, opinion, discourse, ratiocination, are all accidentally depraved by the default of imagination.
>
> (I,1,3,2)

In this determination that both imagination and reason are responsible for delusions, Burton aligned himself with renaissance physician André Du Laurens, as well as the majority of thinkers in his day.[17] (Such an assignment of function reflects the faculty psychology associated with the era and with the emergence of modern psychology. The separate modules of imagination and reason could each become independently impaired.[18]) There remains some unclarity in the roles assigned to reason and imagination, nonetheless.[19] The man who supposes he has no head has a flawed idea, attributed to his imagination, which will in turn affect what else he can believe, for example, whether he needs to wear a hat. This second idea (no hat necessary) will indeed be "depraved," but merely "accidentally" so. If some idea is adopted on the basis of hallucination, subsequent beliefs will be similarly, but only accidentally, inaccurate. This is "perceptual delusion," when mistaken beliefs result from the sensory or phenomenal experience prompted by mistaken perception.[20] Whether or not such "accidental" inferences are to be called delusions, rather than mere illusions, they do seem different from cases where the delusion derives from reasoning which is itself amiss. Some contemporary theorists have defended the rationality of such perceptual delusions, and even analogized every case to these accidental ones. On such a theory, all delusions represent efforts to make sense of anomalous perceptual experiences.[21]

Part 2: Delusional Thought in Today's Mind Science Research

Pathologies of belief, or delusions, have been the subject of much research since the last decade of the twentieth century. Contributors have been philosophers of mind, experimental and cognitive psychologists, and many whose work straddles, and blurs, such disciplinary divisions and boundaries.[22] The question of how to explain and classify such delusional states, and account for puzzling features like their resistance to evidence, has given rise to extensive theorizing and empirical study. While multi-factorial explanatory hypotheses have been increasingly proposed since then, much of this attention initially took the same broad lines of Burton's two-stage, or two-part process of delusion formation. Delusions occur only when there is some further deficiency (of reasoning) added to an aberrant perceptual experience, on this analysis. The recognition that delusions may stem from deficits or damage affecting two separate aspects of cognition have prompted particular attention.

Questions about delusional thought processes presently being explored, each anticipated in the *Anatomy* are: (1) how delusions are to be understood in relation to other cognitive states, particularly beliefs and imaginings, and (2) their causal antecedents. Each question awaits a definitive answer, and each is the source of a range of theories and conjectures.

Delusions in Relation to Beliefs and Imaginings

Two present-day hypotheses, against which Burton's account of the relation between imagination and delusion can be examined, are Andy Egan's hybrid notion of "bimagining," and the identification of delusions as imaginings put forward by Gregory Currie and colleagues. The status of "bimaginings" (part belief, part imagining), has been ascribed to delusional thoughts on the grounds that about the objects (or content), of their delusions, subjects neither straightforwardly believe nor straightforwardly imagine. Thus, "delusional subjects are in states that play a role in their cognitive economies that is in some respects like that of a standard-issue, stereotypical belief that P and in other respects like that of a standard-issue, stereotypical imagining that P."[23] Egan reasons to this conclusion about delusions because their typical *circumscription* (i.e., except in verbal behavior, they are only weakly behavior-guiding), and *evidence-independence*, makes them unlike paradigmatic beliefs (more circumscribed and evidence-dependent) and yet also unlike paradigmatic imaginings, that are less circumscribed and evidence-independent. As a characterization of all delusions, this may be incomplete, since these are at best typical features.[24] But that aside, Egan also points to a methodological presumption required for his account. We must suppose that, as he says, belief and imagining roles are not "package deals" that would preclude such admixtures.[25]

Burton's Aristotelian faculty psychology is a forerunner of today's functionalist representational theories of mind. Representations are the discrete, Fodorian modules that Egan calls "packages" of content, present in the mind in some functionally appropriate way. While sharing content, separate cognitive states such as beliefs, desires and imaginings are distinguished functionally in terms of their differing causal interactions with the outside world and other mental states and processes. In the *Anatomy*, a separated functional role is similarly recognized for each of imagination and reason in respect to delusional phenomena. (Burton's model is renaissance physician André Du Laurens, on this point: "Seeing … that *one of these faculties may be hurt without the other*, we must believe that every one of them hath his particular place" [Du Laurens 1599:80, emphasis added].)

To understand how delusions might nonetheless be hybrids between imagining and believing in the way Egan proposes, however, we may turn to the work of Currie and his colleagues. On traditional, "doxastic" notions, delusions are beliefs, or belief-like. Countering this assumption, these researchers have proposed that delusional thoughts are imaginings, *mistakenly identified as beliefs by their confused subject.*[26] The primary basis for identifying something as an imagined thought is that it is experienced as the outcome of our will, or agency, it is argued, and loss of the capacity to distinguish imaginings is related to a more general loss of a sense of agency toward these mental contents. In this "meta-cognitive" account, the deluded person imagines, rather than believing, a delusional proposition P (while at the same time mistakenly believing that he believes P). A characterization of what is involved in imagining as distinct from believing is analyzed this way:

> [W]hen we imagine something, we do not cease to believe things that are inconsistent with what we imagine, and we do not feel any pressure to resolve clashes between what we believe and what we imagine. Rather beliefs inconsistent with the imagining move temporarily into the background; they are not available as premises in inferences that involve the imagining but are available as premises in inferences that do not. ... imaginings are not apt to be revised in the light of evidence; the whole point of imagining is to enable us to engage with scenarios that we know to be non-actual.
>
> (Currie and Jureidini 2004: 160)

Put in these terms, we can see that Burton's "hurt and misaffected" imagination might be construed as one *unable to recognize and abide by* these respective inferential constraints and freedoms. That one of reason's functions is to recognize and distinguish imagined objects from real ones is evident in a passage that would have been known to Burton. We do not *fear a painted lion*, Du Laurens had explained, because our reason is accustomed to distinguish between the feigned [false] images of the Imagination and the actual objects represented to common sense ("having beheld a painted Lion, it perceiveth that it is not a thing to be feared, and at the same time, joining itself unto reason, doth confirm and make bold" [Du Laurens 1599:75]). With this Laurentian conception of reason's incapacity, likely to have shaped Burton's own reasoning, we can see grounds to name the resulting delusions instances of bimagination along Egan's lines. The function of imagining is distinct from that of believing in the normal case. But delusions reflect *dysfunction*. Then, the imagination is in some way unable to recognize and carry out its normal activities. The ability to distinguish the painted lion as a "feigned" image is a part of normal functioning that has been lost.

Similar claims to these have been developed in relation to disorders resulting in verbal hallucination, hypothesized as a hybrid intentional state lying *somewhere between thinking and perceiving*, or even between remembering and imagining. Encompassing phenomenological disturbances are said to "weaken the boundaries between intentional state types" (Ratcliffe and Wilkinson 2017). Burton is sparing in his account of the flaw or deficiency that occurs when, as he says "our reason is over-ruled, Will precipitated." But this kind of dysfunctional confusion seems one possible interpretation. Colin McGinn offers another very similar description focused on the likely consequence of such a flaw: "the delusional subject has something *wrong* with the way he forms beliefs ... [H]is irrationality consists in letting his beliefs be driven by what is merely imaginary, since images are the wrong *kind* of thing to base beliefs on"(McGinn 2004:115–116).

Both the first idea of a compromised capacity to distinguish one's imaginings from one's beliefs and the suggestion that reason ceases to discern which kinds of thing beliefs should be based on fit Burton's account of delusional thinking. It also fits his insistence that in the thrall of "fond conceits," the melancholic might be misled, granting his fancies a validity, or prominence, that careful attention to their grounds, *and less fondness for them*, would be sufficient to unseat. That we can be mistaken in, and misled by, the objects of our imagining, Burton whole-heartedly accepts: the ungrounded fears he so often cites as symptoms of melancholy concern imagined or imaginary objects. (Burton's emphasis on the power of the imagination to induce or impede healing suggests another kind of misapprehension. Not always maladaptive, this occurs when the person himself is the witting or unwitting target of the imagination's effects. Although not dealt with here, this is a central element of the *Anatomy*.)

On the hypotheses of Currie and his colleagues, imagining cannot be properly *recognized* by the person entertaining delusions, while on Burton's account, the disabled imagination cannot be supervised and curbed by reason. The idea of a compromised capacity to distinguish between imaginings and beliefs tracks, and seems to be complemented by, Burton's analysis of the disordered imagination marking severe Melancholy. When he speaks of the way Reason becomes powerless to monitor and check a runaway imagination, the incapacity is an issue of control – we know we should but cannot stop or help ourselves from succumbing to it. Arguably though, the failure of reason to curb unfettered imagination – a familiar, and time-honored, if imprecise, metaphor – loses little when reformulated as absence of (a sense of) control. An inability to *distinguish believing from imagining* would also preclude the application of the constraints customarily employed for belief acquisition and maintenance. These normal constraints have been described by researchers in terms of a combination of working memory and executive processes of inhibition. The processes involved would thus include assessment of competing hypotheses that could explain the same phenomena, together with inhibition of the imperatives of "observational adequacy" (when seeing is believing), explanatory adequacy (it makes sense) and conservatism (it requires minimal adjustment of any other beliefs).[27]

Those who are not so seriously affected with melancholy have it within their power to resist. They do not always do so. They neglect the many sensible, practical actions derived from attention to daily habits; the solitary charms of melancholy get the better of them, or they are dealt incapacitating blows by the vicissitudes of life. The person *forming* a delusion may willfully turn from evidence challenging her opinion, avoiding those who disagree, hastening to draw conclusions while knowing that speed can be unreliable, or willfully over-generalizing, aware that it will jeopardize accuracy. And some evidence from those with delusions confirms this self-control model. On the other hand, first-person accounts of the phenomenology of full-blown delusional thinking indicate that once a delusion is formed, it sometimes presents itself as so uncontrovertibly correct, convincing or plausible, that nothing can unseat it.[28]

Causal Antecedents

Burton's emphasis on Reason's deficiencies in cases of severe, delusional disorder finds considerable support in contemporary theorizing. Presently the most influential theoretical explanatory model of delusion hypothesizes two distinct deficiencies. Aberrant, confusing or alarming perceptual experience is one. But only combined with flawed induction can aberrant experiences explain the formation and maintenance of delusions.[29] Several aspects of the details of this model follow Burton's conjectures in the passage quoted earlier.[30]

Most importantly, two factors are involved. A two-way interaction explains how the anomalous experience and reasoning about it first form, and then maintain, delusional states.[31] Like Burton, two-factor theorists propose that only after and as a response to the first factor does the cognitive defect convert the anomalous experience into a delusional belief, making up a uni-directional causal sequence. This theoretical model hypothesizes some form of brain damage or dysfunction, which may manifest itself in felt experience, as the first factor. (Likely experiences have been postulated to include heightened perceptual awareness, states of arousal, and the unexpected presence or absence of feelings of familiarity.[32, 33]) The second element, corresponding to Burton's (and Avicenna's) corrupted reason, is a deficiency within reasoning.

The demand for a second factor argues that the presence of these experiences (the first factor) may be necessary but cannot be sufficient to explain delusion formation, for there are other discomforting or anomalous experiences that do not result in delusional states. Like Burton and the ancient medical writers he cites, who speak of an additional flaw in Reason itself, this second factor in delusion formation has usually been understood as a cognitive feature affecting a person's belief formation.[34, 35] In ordinary belief formation on this analysis, experience triggers a plausible ("candidate") belief, which is subject to a process of critical review ("belief fixation") in light of other information. When delusions form, it is as the result of deficiency or dysfunction in this process of critical review.

Attempts to account for the second factor have included bias in the style of attribution (explanations of experiences and events). An "externalizing" attribution style, that ascribes negative events to other people rather than to circumstances, has been proposed to partially explain persecutory delusions, for example.[36] Similar claims have been made for the inferential habit known as the jumping-to-conclusions bias, and its allied tendency to ignore alternative explanations.[37] A distorting inclination to privilege the "seeing is believing" impact of the immediate experience (known as "observational adequacy") over as little as possible disturbing the subject's other beliefs has also been hypothesized.[38]

Construed as (second factor) defects of inference along these lines, delusional belief formation shows close parallels with more commonplace errors of judgment. Normal and non-delusional reasoners exhibit each of the irrationalities described in this two-factor account: they make unwarranted inferences of every kind, and succumb to assessments that are biased and overly hasty.[39] The normal reasoner's irrationalities are customarily assumed to allow remedy through attention, effort and care, while the delusional person's reasoning errors indicate dysfunction or incapacity that, at least in application to the phenomena comprising the first factor, *cannot* be overcome at all, or can be overcome only with great difficulty. If the delusional person's defect merely calls for a greater effort than the normal reasoner's, then in one respect, although he may need to try harder, and even seek help in countering his irrational tendencies, the deluded person shares a continuum with more normal reasoners. The difference marking his or her reasoning deficiency may lie merely with the presence of the first factor which affects it, or with a greater degree of bias and distortion. (These ideas require us to accept that delusional and non-delusional cases are quantitatively, rather than qualitatively distinguishable. Even normal irrationalities are sufficiently sub-personal and extensive to belie the part played there by attention, effort and care, it is sometimes suggested.

If what we can and cannot do were unaffected by what we fondly think is involved in making an effort, however, the second-factor irrationalities of the delusional patient and the illogic of normal folk may be not merely continuous, but *indistinguishable* – undermining the basis for so construing the second factor. Burton had no doubt that attention, effort and care could and would make a difference in relation to normal reasoning, however. It is only in severe, intractable Melancholy that such capabilities are lost.)

Two-factor theorizing was developed for the subset of delusions associated with brain damage or disease, and may be limited in its application.[40] Its breadth and flexibility are notable, however, potentially accommodating variations in the first factor (including whether it permits subjective awareness); in the degree to which the two factors are linked, which may be more or less elaborated, and semantically attenuated; and in the range of illogical and biased forms of reasoning comprising the second factor.[41] The capacity of two-factor theorizing to explain the diversity among delusional states also extends to variations in the assignment of relative explanatory burden. A more alarming first factor may take little beyond the normal degree of inferential error to result in a delusion, whereas matched with more profound inferential deficits, less salient experiences might have the same effect. Combined with the widely held presumption that delusions form a distinct medical class, this breadth and flexibility seem to position two-factor theorizing to apply to a diversity of delusional states, extending even to those referred to in Burton's abbreviated cases.[42]

The limited and usually second-hand clinical tales offered in the *Anatomy* are difficult to categorize in any but the broadest terms, it should be added, and give little indication of the types of delusions they might be. A small group of delusions has received attention in contemporary research thus far. Of those, neither delusions of misidentification, such as the much-studied Capgras, or of Alien Control, are represented in the *Anatomy*. Persecutory delusions, another subject of recent study, do appear. Even so, the examples in the *Anatomy* are very sparing in their details. It is difficult to know whether some of these cases involve delusional systems, for example, with elaborate webs of belief with coherent internal logic, or fixed, single-themed (monothematic) delusions that leave the rest of cognitive functioning intact and unaffected. Nor can we tell whether these develop slowly, by recognizably inferential steps, or arrive full-blown, out of momentary perceptual experience; or the extent to which they are detached from the rest of the person's psychic life and behavior, or fade and reappear according to the course of recurrent or episodic conditions. None of these variations can be excluded from the case records Burton cites, but nor are they helpfully illuminated.

Today's two-factor analyses employ richer and more complete cases.[43] Such material shows that delusions vary greatly in their degree of elaboration, only sometimes taking the form of explanations offered for aberrant experiences. At other times, they resemble the kind of "endorsements" that we associate with the perceptual experience that is the basis of belief about the world around us and confidently accepted at face value. Once prompted by the initiating and content-fixing element of aberrant experience, two-factor theorizing has proposed a range of ways the formation and adoption of a delusional idea occurs, depending on the type of first factor involved. Because an aberrant perceptual experience may fully exhaust the representational content of a delusion, it has been pointed out, merely taking hallucinatory experience at face value and endorsing it may be sufficient to produce a delusion. Such perceptual delusions derived from hallucination certainly differ from the more elaborate processes of hypothesis construction and confirmation implicated in other delusional reasoning depicted by two-factor theorizing.[44] And so do delusions apparently prompted as groundless intuitions from unrelated perceptual experience.[45]

Burton sides with Avicenna in controversies over the causal sequence by which delusional thinking occurs: the disease is "first in Imagination, and afterwards in reason," but the "hurt and misaffected" imagination initiates the sequence (1,1,3,2:164–5). And two-factor theorizing also proposes a fixed, uni-directional causal sequence: only after and as a response to the first factor does the reasoning defect convert the anomalous experience (or data) into a delusional thought, or assertion.[46] This sequence has been expanded, and a picture of two-way interaction proposed to account for how delusional states are maintained.[47] Thus, although the initial formation of the delusion results from a fixed causal order (from neurological defect, to anomalous experience, to delusional belief formation), the interaction between distorted belief and *continuing misperception* serves to explain why delusional notions are not revised, and are instead tenaciously held.[48] Burton's claims and those of the authorities he cites are not incompatible with this multi-directional sequence. Without the *initially* disturbed imagining, the claim is, the sequence would not occur.

We learn few details about how reason is deficient in the two-factor theories described in the *Anatomy*; Burton resorts to metaphor. Yet his overall sense of the way reason can be overcome by an unruly imagination, or weak will, seems to concur with these contemporary two-factor theories. And far from being distinctive to the deluded reasoner, aberrant reasoning patterns, bias and misapprehension are in the *Anatomy* accepted as an unavoidable part of our human legacy. Whether or not as the result of the distorting effect of our passions, as Burton thought, bias and error are entirely normal ways of apprehending the world and processing our thoughts. Delusions, in this depiction, are continuous with more ordinary error-based misapprehensions.

This gradualist approach to second-factor theorizing that places delusions on a continuum with normal cognitive processing has its detractors. In a recent analysis, Philip Gerrans has argued for a stronger division between delusions and more normal misconceptions and errors, rejecting as inadequate the doxastic assumptions of the two-factor theorizing described above. In that theorizing, he explains, delusional and normal belief fixation alike mirror the way, on the epistemic model of scientific hypothesis-making, we are thought to understand the world. According to the alternative account offered by Gerrans, however, delusions are produced by, and locked into, the default network engaged in the process of providing "subjectively adequate default response to salient information" (Gerrans 2014: 115). Rather than treating particular thoughts or narrative fragments as empirical hypotheses, on analogy with the scientific approach employed by normal reasoners, reduced dorsolateral activity in the deluded reasoner's brain *prevents* "decontextualized supervision." The critical evaluation of the thought as a descriptive statement that may or may not be consistent with other beliefs and relevant evidence is an operation that the subject is unable to undertake. The thought is thus confined within its default system fortress. From there, depending on the nature and degree of the dysfunction in the dorsolateral region, it is accepted and conserved, and may go on to structure the deluded person's subsequent thinking and behavior. (The hypoactivation in right dorsolateral areas widely believed implicated in delusion is offered as support for Gerrans's analysis. The dorsolateral system provides decontextualized supervision for the default system. When that system is lesioned or hypoactive, on this hypothesis, "activity in the default system is unsupervised," resulting in the generation and elaboration of delusional thoughts.)

This is not the only alternative to the standard two-factor theorizing described above. Important work has hypothesized that prediction-error is the source of delusions, for example.[49] However, Gerrans's account has particular bearing for us since it locates the problem within the same default system to which Burton's faculty of imagination can be shown to largely correspond. Moreover, like Burton's, Gerrans also puts forward a two-factor account. A default system thought or narrative fragment is triggered by a perceptual or sensory anomaly (the first factor). As an imaginative state not subject to metacognitive supervision, it is uncritically accepted and employed within subsequent cognitive activity. (Gerrans uses the term "incorporation" to describe this process of uncritical acceptance and employment.) How to account for what goes wrong is where Gerrans differs from other two-factor theorists. This is not merely a case of extremely biased and faulty supervision of the default thought, the required supervisory decontextualized processing system is broken, and cannot function. In support of this claim, Gerrans points to some preliminary evidence that in patients with schizophrenic delusions, the relevant dorsolateral circuitry is hypoactive.[50] More generally, Gerrans's focus on deficiencies in the default system is identified with some findings linked to schizophrenia. Even when attending to external stimuli and directed tasks, those diagnosed with schizophrenia exhibit greater levels of default system activity. From this it is concluded that the default network system is in this group "hyper-connected and hyperactive" (Whitfield-Gabrieli et al., 2009).[51] This finding, that the default mode cannot be "turned down," resonates with both Gerrans's hypotheses, and with Burton's repeated insistence that the imagination is somehow overly active in those afflicted with melancholy.

At first sight, the success of cognitive therapy and the hypothesis-testing described in first person accounts of successful self-analysis by those who have been afflicted with delusions appear to preclude Gerrans's alternative understanding of how delusions are acquired. Yet the fact that delusions sometimes remit in the face of hypothetical reasoning does not show that they *originate* as the result of (erroneous) hypothetical, empirical science-style reasoning, Gerrans (rightly) insists.[52] For several reasons, however, Burton would diverge from Gerrans in rejecting the hypothesis-testing model of how delusions are initially acquired. First, he acknowledges that bias and other reasoning faults are present in non-delusional reasoners to a lesser degree. Indeed, because of the spell cast by the imagination, they are an endless temptation and hazard for all reasoners. In addition, as we saw, his account of how friends can help with delusions includes a process of rational persuasion and analysis which (loosely) follows the epistemic model analogous to processes of scientific inquiry. But more importantly, Burton's is, for better or worse, a habituation model of severe melancholy. These delusional states are an outcome of the bad cognitive habits of the *akratic* melancholic; they are the dire cost any of us might have to pay for neglecting to monitor the unruly activities of an over-active imagination, and the dangerously intense feelings they engender.

In its broader themes also, the *Anatomy* seems more consonant with the standard two-factor theorizing. Burton stresses the commonality between melancholy as disease and the more normal responses that make us human. With the Stoics, his focus is on the errors and failures of reason, to which we are all heir. The hypothesis-testing model is not wholly his. But more importantly, nor is it wholly complete, since it omits feelings and passions. (The exclusion of emotions from most contemporary models of delusion, which Burton would deplore, has recently been recognized.[53]) He would suppose delusions formed through some combination that included at least three factors: (1) neglected or errant hypothesis-testing, (2) a raging imagination and (3) unregulated passions. We cherish our "fond conceits" and it is those inclinations and feelings that engender and *motivate* the errors and biases in our reasoning.

Note on Delusions and Dreams

Burton accepts a long tradition whereby the imagination produces both delusions and dreams.[54] The link is of special importance since disturbed and troubling dreams are frequently alluded to as symptoms of melancholy.[55] These and all dreams, Burton says, are brought about by "a concourse of bad humors" (I, 2,3,2:250). Elsewhere, he explains further:

> The affections of ... [the] Senses are Sleep and Waking, common to all sensible creatures ... [When] the common sense resteth, the outward senses rest also. [Then] The Phantasie alone is free ... This ligation of Senses, proceeds from an inhibition of spirits, the way being stopped by which they should come; this stopping is caused by the vapours arising out of the stomacke, filling the Nerves, by which the spirits should be conveyed. When these vapours are spent, the passage is open, and the spirits perform their accustomed duties...
>
> (I,1,2,7:153)

Despite its humoral language and presuppositions, this description of dreaming actually corresponds to several aspects of contemporary analyses. Not only is the Imagination the central factor in dreaming, a time-honored position still adhered to by some contemporary thinkers in debates over whether dreams are some form of belief, as the parallels between dreams and delusions in Burton's account match those contemporary analyses, including that of Gerrans. As described in the above passage, sensory functions rest when we dream (in this, it reflects default system functioning), imagination is entirely free, and the "customary duties," which include the supervisory efforts of reason, are temporarily stopped.

In each of these elements, Burton's account corresponds to that offered by Gerrans's portrayal of dreams as an extreme case of hyper-associative default processing. Delusions are not dreams, but "they have some of the properties of 'normal' waking cognition" (Gerrans 2014:69). Dreams and delusions share important properties of default thinking inasmuch as they involve activation of components of a network that "simulates a stream of personally relevant experiences and thoughts *in the absence of actual perceptual input or supervision by decontextualized thought*" (Gerrans 2014: 152–153, emphasis added). There are differences between dreaming and delusional thinking: only in the latter, while the interplay between the default system and normal cognition is compromised, the functioning of the default system remains "embedded in the overall functioning of the mind" in still receiving input from sensory and memory systems. (Gerrans 2014: 151–152). Once we set aside the obvious differences related to Gerrans's more accurate brain science, it seems clear that the emphasis on dreams as default system activity more thoroughly divorced from normal sensory and supervisory functions is not substantially changed in the two accounts. And as we saw earlier, so is the absence or deactivation of the supervisory feature in the case of delusional thinking. Night dreaming, the day dreaming of mind-wandering, and delusional thought processes have similarities in addition to their obvious differences.

In some respects, the two-factor account most closely resembling the *Anatomy*'s is one in which normal supervisory functions are *entirely* dysfunctional or, in Burton's word, "corrupted." That failure may still be a product of cognitive bias, and correspond to scientific methodology (contra Gerrans). Based on the ease with which experiences and events can be imagined, or brought to mind, what is known as the imagination or simulation bias distorts probability judgment about them. And these limitations on imagining may yet be so stringent they entirely *prevent* imagining alternative explanations, rather than merely making it more difficult. The process by which more realistic or plausible hypotheses can be brought to mind may be not merely impaired but broken. Thus, Burton's two-factor account from Avicenna is compatible with present-day standard two-factor theorizing. It need not relinquish the parallels maintained in the *Anatomy* between more normal, flawed reasoning and the errors of the person harboring delusions.

Conclusion

The many tales of apparently delusional misapprehensions and notions in the *Anatomy* correspond loosely to the categories of hallucination and delusion in today's psychology, yet Burton provides us with thin, likely misleading, symptom and case depictions. By contrast, his theoretical account is rich and full of substantive claims, several of which share assumptions and principles with the important recent work on delusional states coming out of contemporary mind sciences. His acceptance of the view that a disordered or deficient imagination is the source of such aberrant thinking is one of these, along with a conception of imagining that corresponds to the default attentional system. The parallels he draws between delusions and dreams are another. And finally, his elaborated two-factor causal analysis, we saw, aligns Burton's to standard models employed within cognitive psychology.

Much of the *Anatomy* is unreliably speculative, with some parts even intentionally misleading. Yet about delusional thinking, Burton offers us ideas that are not only historically illuminating, but coherent, logically grounded and pertinent to ongoing debates within today's mind sciences.

Notes

1 Burton (1577–1640) spent his adult life at Oxford, completing successive editions of *The Anatomy of Melancholy* after the first in 1621. Quoted passages in what follows are from the Third Edition (1628). Except when otherwise noted, italics are in original; Partitions are shown with Roman numbers, followed by Sections, Members and Subsections and page numbers indicated by Arabic ones. For more about Burton's work and times see Gowland 2007, Lund 2010.
2 "Some laughe, weepe, some are mad, some dejected…" (I,3,1,3:402).
3 MacDonald 1981: 155–157.
4 On the relation between melancholy and our present-day mood disorders, see Radden 2003, Varga 2013.
5 Renaissance thinker Timothie Bright makes a clear separation between natural and unnatural forms of the humor. Unnatural sorts of humor, on his account, have been "wholly changed into another nature by an unkindly heat" (Bright 1995: 2).
6 Kramer 2005: 158–171.
7 Themes involving sex, jealousy and religion each play a prominent role in the content of delusions observed in the clinic today. Yet despite the Third Partition devoted to love and religious melancholy, and Burton's seeming recognition that these particular ideas are regular incitements to psychic distress and imbalance, the analysis of these particular forms of melancholy fails to improve on or alter those offered in the first two Partitions. Establishing that these aspects of our lives make us vulnerable to disorder, is the limit of Burton's interest. (For example, of the religious "prophets and dreamers amongst us" he remarks, "whom we persecute with fire and fagot, I thinke the most compendious cure for some of them at least, had beene in Bedlam" [III,4,1,5:395]).
8 I,3,1,3: 402.
9 I,3,1,2: 385.
10 I,3,1,2: 386.
11 On the distinction between monothematic and polythematic delusions, see Davies and Coltheart 2000, Coltheart 2013.
12 See MacDonald 1981:153–154.
13 I,1,3,2:164.
14 This analysis is repeated in the Third Partition, and employed to confirm that love melancholy is appropriately so called. In its sufferer: "both imagination and reason are misaffected, because of his corrupt judgement, and continuall meditation of that which he desires, he may truly be said to be melancholy. If it be violent, or his disease inveterate … both imagination and reason are misaffected, first one, then the other" (III,2,1,2:58).
15 See Bayne and Pacherie 2005, Radden 2000, McKenna 2017.
16 These characteristics of delusional thought are described by Karl Jaspers 1913, but see also Davies and Coltheart 2000.
17 Jackson 1986:90.
18 See Radden 2003, Varga 2013:147–148.
19 Quoting Rhasis the Arabian, Burton at one stage suggests a three-part functional division.

> The first is falsa cognitatio, false conceats and idle thoughts: to misconster and amplify, aggravating everything they conceive or fear; the second is falso cogitate loqui, to talk to themselves or to use inarticulate, incondite voices, speeches, obsolete gestures, and plainly to utter their minds and conceits of their hearts by their words and actions...; the third is to put in practice that which they think or speak.

20 See Bayne and Pacherie 2005, also Radden 2000:26–27. Delusional perception, by contrast, occurs when an apparently normal perceptual experience triggers a delusional idea.

21 This is the one-factor account, whereby delusion is an hypothesis designed to explain unusual perceptual phenomena and developed through the operation of normal cognitive processes (Maher 1999). The misapprehensions that result from hallucination differ only from delusions proper in that the former stem from experiences that are more accessible to conscious awareness, and identified as perceptual experiences. Or, as it has been put: "there is nothing irrational about forming false beliefs on the basis of illusions and hallucinations" (McGinn 2004:115).

22 See Garrety and Hemsley 1994, Davies and Coltheart 2000, Bayne and Pacherie 2005, Broome and Bortolotti 2009, Aimola Davies and Davies 2009, Broome and McGuire 2009, Bortolotti 2010, Egan 2009, Radden 2000, Young 2011.

23 Egan 2009:268.

24 Radden 2000.

25 Egan 2009.

26 Currie 2000, Currie and Ravenscroft 2002, Broome and McGuire 2009.

27 Aimola Davies and Davies 2009.

28 See Radden 2000: 100–108.

29 Davies, Coltheart, Langdon, and Breen 2009.

30 One of these is that although it has also been proffered to explain delusions as they are embedded in syndromal clusters (psychosis), as well as diagnostic disorder categories, two-factor theorizing has been applied to delusions regarded as free-standing symptoms, along the lines of Burton's symptoms-oriented approach. See Fletcher and Frith 2009).

31 Young 2011, Fletcher and Frith 2009.

32 Broome and McGuire 2009: 283–284.

33 Aberrations of perception are also the starting point of prediction error hypotheses, which rest on the idea of a mismatch between prior expectations understood in Bayesian terms and such immediate experience (Uhlhaas and Mishara 2007, Mishara and Corlett 2009).

34 Davies and Coltheart 2000.

35 Counting factors slightly differently, others have separated the process that leads from the initial deficit or experience to the full state of belief acceptance, proposing instead a three-stage framework that includes hypothesis construction (Aimola Davies and Davies 2009).

36 Bentall 2003.

37 Stone and Young 1997, Freeman, Bentall and Garety 2008.

38 Stone and Young 1997.

39 See Kahneman 2011.

40 This has been recognized, see Coltheart 2013.

41 Aimola Davies and Davies 2009:315.

42 For that range, see Radden 2000.

43 Arguably, much of this research still lacks an adequately rich place-setting in terms of context and natural history.

44 When the Capgras patient proceeds from the sense of something strange about the look of his spouse to "Someone must be pretending to be my wife," the delusional state encompasses what has been described as an *explanation*, as distinct from mere *endorsement* (Aimola Davies and Davies 2009:290–291).

45 In some clinical writing there are also what are known as delusional perceptions or delusional percepts: when some idea or train of ideas, accompanied by a sense of significance and meaning, is abruptly and unaccountably triggered by everyday, unexceptional, perceptual experience. (This is the German *Wahneinfall* [delusional intuition].)

46 Perceptions, sensations and all manner of subjective feeling are affected by expectations so that these separate cognitive and perceptual elements merge. Unusual perceptual experiences of patients and their sometimes bizarre beliefs have been said to be "part of the same core abnormality," identified as a disturbance in error-dependent updating of inferences and beliefs about the world, so that "it is possible to understand these symptoms in terms of a disturbed hierarchical Bayesian framework, *without recourse to separate considerations of experience and belief.*" Recent computational models of perception and learning "suggest that the same fundamental mechanism (Bayesian inference) by which a model of the world is updated by prediction errors, applies to both perception and belief" (Fletcher and Frith 2009:01, my emphasis).

47 Young 2008, 2011.

48 As Young notes, in accounting for why delusions fail to develop in other conditions that seemingly start with parallel deficits (patients with bilateral lesions to the ventromedial frontal lobes): even if other conditions begin with damage of the kind hypothesized for the delusional patient, only in the delusional case (of the Capgras delusion) are the belief and the experience mutually sustaining in the manner of a feedback loop (Young 2011).

49 See Fletcher and Frith 2009.

50 Gerrans 2014:148.

51 This study examined the default network in patients diagnosed with early phases of schizophrenia and their young first-degree relatives, using functional MRI while patients and controls alternated between rest and performance of working memory tasks. The controls exhibited task-related suppression of activation in the default network, including medial prefrontal cortex (MPFC) and posterior cingulate cortex/precuneus. Patients and relatives exhibited significantly reduced task-related suppression in MPFC, and these reductions remained after controlling for performance. Also, during rest and task, patients and relatives exhibited abnormally high functional connectivity within the default network and the magnitudes of default network connectivity during rest and task correlated with psychopathology in the patients. The study concluded that "hyperactivation" or reduced task-related suppression of default regions and hyperconnectivity of the default network likely contribute to, and enhance the risk for, thought disturbances in schizophrenia. (Whitfield-Gabrieli et al. 2009).

52 Gerrans 2014:159.

53 See Ratcliffe and Wilkinson 2017.

54 For example, Du Laurens makes the connection between dreams and delusions: it "happeneth all alike" to melancholike persons as to those which dream,

he says, and "dreames have recourse until the imagination as well as melancholie" (Du Laurens 1599:99).

55 On the "terrible dreames" afflicting the melancholic, see I,3,1,1: 383; also I,3,2,2:411.

Bibliography

Aimola Davies, A. and Davies, M. Davies, 2009. Explaining pathologies of belief. In *Psychiatry as Cognitive Neuroscience: Philosophical Perspectives.* Edited by Matthew Broome and Lisa Bortolotti. Oxford: Oxford University Press, 285–326.

American Psychiatric Association. 2013. *Diagnostic and Statistical Manual of Mental Disorders.* 5th Edition. Washington, DC: American Psychiatric Association.

Bayne, T., and Pacherie, E. 2005. In defence of the doxastic conception of delusions. *Mind and Language* 20:163–188.

Bentall, R. 2003. *Madness Explained.* London: Penguin.

Berrios, G. 2011. *Preface to Diseases of the Imagination and Imaginary Disease in the Early Modern Period.* Edited by Y. Haskell. Turnhout: Brepols; xv–xxiii.

Bortolotti, L. 2010. *Delusions and Other Irrational Beliefs.* Oxford: Oxford University Press.

Bright, T. 1995. *A Treatise of Melancholy.* New York: The Classics of Psychiatry & Behavioral Sciences Library.

Broome, M., and Bortolotti, L. 2009. *Psychiatry as Cognitive Neuroscience: Philosophical Perspectives.* Oxford: Oxford University Press.

Broome, M., and McGuire, P.K. 2009. Imagining and delusions. In *Persecutory Delusions: Assessment, Theory and Treatment.* Edited by D. Freeman, R. Bentall, and P. Garety. Oxford: Oxford University Press.

Burton, R. 1632/1989–2000. *The Anatomy of Melancholy*, vol 6. Edited by Thomas Faulkner, Nicolas Kiessling, and Rhonda Blair. Vols. I–III: text; vols. IV–VI: commentary by J.B. Bamborough and Martin Dodsworth. Oxford: Oxford University Press.

Coltheart, M. 2013. On the distinction between monothematic and polythematic delusions. *Mind and Language* 28:103–112.

Currie, G. 2000. Imagination, delusion and hallucination. In *Pathologies of Belief*, edited by M. Coltheart and M. Davies. Oxford: Blackwell, 167–182.

Currie, G., and Jureidini, J. 2004. Narrative and coherence. *Mind and Language* 19:409–427.

Currie, G., and Ravenscroft, I. 2002. *Recreative Imagination.* Oxford: Oxford University Press.

Delusion and Self-Deception: Affective and Motivational Influences on Belief Formation. Edited by Tim Bayne and Jordi Fernandez. New York: Psychology Press, 187–225.

Davies, M., et al. 2001a. Monothematic delusions: towards a two-factor account. *Philosophy, Psychiatry and Psychology* 8:133–158.

Davies, M., and Coltheart, M. 2000. Introduction: pathologies of belief. *Mind and Language* 15(1):1–46.

Davies, M., Coltheart, M., Langdon, R., and Breen, N. 2001b. Monothematic delusions: towards a two-factor account. *Philosophy, Psychiatry, & Psychology* 8(2):133–158.

Du Laurens, A. 1599/1938. *A Discourse of the Preservation of the Sight: Of Melancholike Diseases; of Rheumes, and of Old Age*. Edited by M. Andreas Laurentius, translated by Richard Surphlet. London: Humphrey Milford, Oxford University Press, Amen House, Warwick Square, E.C.

Egan, A. 2009. Imagination, delusion and self-deception. In *Delusion and Self-Deception: Affective and Motivational Influences on Belief Formation*, edited by T. Bayne and J. Fernandez. New York: Psychology Press, 263–280.

Freeman, D., Bentall, R., and Garety, P. (eds). 2008. *Persecutory Delusions: Assessment, Theory and Treatment*. Oxford: Oxford University Press.

Fletcher, P.C., and Frith, C.D. (2009). Perceiving is believing: a Bayesian approach to explaining the positive symptoms of schizophrenia. *Nature Reviews Neuroscience* 10(1):48–58.

Garrety, P., and Hemsley, D.R. 1994. *Delusions: Investigations into the Psychology of Delusional Reasoning*. Oxford: Oxford University Press.

Gerrans, P. 2014. *The Measure of Madness: Philosophy of Mind, Cognitive Neuroscience, and Delusional Thought*. Cambridge: MIT Press.

Gowland, A. 2007. *The Worlds of Renaissance Melancholy: Robert Burton in Context*. Cambridge: Cambridge University Press.

Jackson, S. 1986. *Melancholia and Depression: From Hippocratic Times to Modern Times*. London: Yale University Press.

Jaspers, K. 1963. *General Psychopathology*. Toronto: University of Toronto Press.

Johnson, S. 1893. *Letters*. Edited by G.B. Hill. Oxford: Oxford University Press. Vol 1.

Kahneman, D. 2011. *Thinking Fast and Slow*. New York: Penguin.

Kramer, P. 2005. *Against Depression*. New York: Viking.

Liao, Shen-yi, and Gendler, Tamar 2020. Imagination. In *The Stanford Encyclopedia of Philosophy* (Summer 2020 Edition), Edward N. Zalta (ed.), https://plato.stanford.edu/archives/sum2020/entries/imagination/

Lund, M. 2010. *Melancholy, Medicine and Religion in Early Modern England: Reading the Anatomy of Melancholy*. Cambridge: Cambridge University Press.

Macdonald, M. 1981. *Mystical Bedlam: Madness, Anxiety, and Healing in Seventeenth-Century England*. Cambridge: Cambridge University Press.

Maher, B. 1999. Anomalous experience in everyday life. *The Monist* 82:547–570.

McGinn, C. 2004. *Mindsight: Image, Dream, Meaning*. Cambridge, MA: Harvard University Press.

McKenna, P. 2017. *Delusions: Understanding the Un-understandable*. Cambridge: Cambridge University Press.

Mishara, A.L., and Corlett, P. 2009. Are delusions biologically adaptive? Salvaging the doxastic shear pin. *Behavioral and Brain Sciences* 32:530–531.

Radden, J. (ed). 2000. *The Nature of Melancholy: From Aristotle to Kristeva*. New York: Oxford University Press.

Radden, J. 2003. Is this dame melancholy? Equating depression and melancholia. *Psychiatry, Philosophy and Psychology* 10(1):37–52.

Ratcliffe, M., and Wilkinson, S. 2017. *Verbal Hallucinations, Emotions, and the Interpersonal World*. Cambridge, MA: MIT Press.

Stone, Tony, and Young, Andrew W. 1997. Delusions and brain injury: the philosophy and psychology of belief. *Mind and Language* 12(3–4):327–364.

Tilmouth, C. 2005. Burton's "Turning Picture": argument and anxiety in the *Anatomy of Melancholy*. *Review of English Studies* 56:524–549.

Uhlhaas, P.J., and Mishara, A.L. 2007. Perceptual anomalies in schizophrenia: integrating phenomenology and cognitive neuroscience. *Schizophrenia Bulletin* 33:142–156.

Varga, S. 2013. From melancholia to depression: ideas on a possible continuity. *Philosophy, Psychiatry, and Psychology* 20:141–155.

Whitfield-Gabrieli, S., et al. 2009. Hyperactivity and hyperconnectivity of the default network in schizophrenia and in first-degree relatives of persons with schizophrenia. *Proceedings of the National Academy of Sciences* 106:1279–1284.

Wright, T. 1986. *The Passions of the Mind in General*. Edited by W.W. Newbold. New York and London: Garland.

Young, G. 2011. Beliefs, experiences, and misplaced being: an interactionist account of delusional misidentification. *Phenomenology and the Cognitive Sciences* 10:195–215.

Young, G. 2008. Capgras delusion: an interactionist model. *Consciousness and Cognition* 17:863–876.

Part II

Varieties of Everyday Delusion

5 Meaning and Delusion

Rick Bellaar and Jasper Feyaerts

Introduction

Delusions are typically formulated in terms of knowing rather than believing.[1] Since claiming 'I know' typically entails that I believe, the delusional 'I know' could be considered consistent with the dominant doxastic view that delusions are (wrong) beliefs.[2] However, such doxasticism about delusions has received substantial criticism.[3] For example, it has been argued that the ways in which beliefs can be irrational are contingent and that such irrationality is not specific to delusions.[4] As an alternative to the doxastic view, some philosophers have proposed that the irrationality that does specifically mark (primary) delusions consists of conflicts with Wittgensteinian objective certainties.[5] Such objective certainties are norms that are constitutive of knowledge. On such a view, the delusional 'I know' is applied to that which logically *cannot* function as knowledge rather than to that which empirically *does* not function as knowledge. (Delusional) speech that conflicts with such norms is therefore not merely contingently irrational, but necessarily so, setting apart delusional irrationality from everyday contingently irrational beliefs.[6]

Such a proposed conflict with objective certainties has led others to claim that (pre-)delusional states involve the loss of these certainties.[7] However, claims of lost objective certainties in delusions have also received criticism: it has been argued that objective certainties cannot be compromised in delusion,[8] and that the disintegration of ordinary intentionality resulting from such a loss more adequately describes dementia, catatonic or disorganized conditions rather than delusion.[9] Instead, it has been argued that the delusional use of 'I know' is either nonsensical or has the form of avowals.[10]

The aim of the current chapter is to focus on the latter alternative and to show more specifically *how* delusional language can be thought to consist of *meaningful avowals*[11] of *knowledge*. We will proceed by analogy with feelings of unreality. Such feelings may frequently co-occur with or precede

DOI: 10.4324/9781003288992-8

delusions and have themselves sometimes been conceptualized in terms of a loss of objective certainty.[12] However, if delusions cannot involve lost objective certainties, it is warranted to question whether co-occurring feelings of unreality can. In this chapter, we will see how expressions of feelings of unreality can be conceptualized as avowals that *presuppose* objective certainty rather than its *loss*. Conceived in this manner, feelings of unreality can provide a model – rather than an enabling condition – for understanding delusions. We will pursue this line of thought and see how delusional language can be understood as avowals of pathological knowledge.[13]

Unreality – Ratcliffe

Ratcliffe (2013) follows Jaspers in analyzing our various forms of intentionality (including knowing, doubting and believing) in terms of an experienced 'sense of reality'. On Ratcliffe's view, the *function* of this experienced sense of reality is to enable our different ways of relating to reality, that is, to enable different *modes of intentionality*:

> A sense of what it is to be 'not there' depends upon a sense of what it is to be 'there'. More generally, a sense of what it is to be 'not real' depends upon a sense of what it is to be 'real'. So other kinds of intentional state, such as imagining, remembering, anticipating, doubting, and so forth (all of which incorporate a sense of these distinctions) equally depend upon the experienced sense of reality.[14]

A wide array of intentional states are argued to rely on this experienced sense of reality, but for our purposes here, it suffices to note that at least epistemic notions such as doubt, belief and knowledge are said to logically presuppose it. These forms of epistemic intentionality are claimed to be *enabled* by this sense of reality: without such a sense, we would not be able to have this *kind* of intentionality. Functionally then, in enabling doubt, belief (whether false and true), and knowledge, the sense of reality thus posited can be thought to align with notions found in the (mostly phenomenological) literature such as 'reality contact',[15] 'frame conditions',[16] 'the ontological framework',[17] 'common sense',[18] 'natural self-evidence',[19] 'the natural attitude',[20] or the 'sense of reality'.[21]

Ratcliffe[22] and Varga[23] have also explicitly connected the (loss of the) sense of reality with (the loss of) Wittgensteinian (1974) 'objective certainty'. According to Ratcliffe, feelings of unreality involve disturbed certainties, resulting in the disintegration of ordinary modes of intentionality, which are in turn appealed to in order to render delusions intelligible. Certainties too make possible the meaningful employment of epistemic notions such as doubt, knowledge and belief. It is therefore not surprising that authors such as Ratcliffe (2008, 2015, 2017) take the notion of a sense of reality to be intricately related to the notion of objective certainty (also: 'hinges' or 'framework propositions').

> [According to Jaspers] 'belief' presupposes a different kind of confidence or certainty. This same position can be arrived at through a consideration of themes in Ludwig Wittgenstein's later writings.[24]
>
> It is ... arguable that Wittgenstein is not discussing 'propositions' in any familiar sense of the term and that his framework propositions might add up to what I refer to as the sense of reality.[25]
>
> Thus some 'hinge propositions' are integral to our sense of reality, to our sense of what it is to be present, the case, real.[26]

Elaborating on the work of Ratcliffe, Varga (2012a, 2012b) puts succinctly the connection between the two notions:

> The idea [is] that the characteristic feelings of 'unreality' are connected to a diminished sense of 'realness,' which – rather than being a question of belief or propositional content – is located on the level of a primordial and pre-intentional relation to the world.[27]

Accordingly, when our everyday experiential sense of reality is diminished, feelings of unreality arise. For Ratcliffe and Varga, the relevance of this sense of reality to the psychopathology of delusion is that its loss – manifested in reported feelings of unreality in (pre-)delusional atmosphere[28] – provides the *enabling* condition of primary delusions:

> The claim is not simply that delusional atmosphere [including experiences of unreality] causes delusional beliefs to arise. Rather, primary delusions are intelligible only in the context of such an experience. By analogy, a checkmate situation would not be intelligible outside of a chess game. Thus, to understand the delusion, we also need to understand the more enveloping experience in which it is embedded.
>
> (Ratcliffe 2017, p 109)

We see that whereas a sense of reality is an enabling condition for believing and doubting, and the like, the loss of the sense of reality is said to enable delusions. As such, pointing to this loss supposedly helps us to understand *how delusions are intelligibly possible*. Precisely because such a loss entails a breakdown of ordinary modes of intentionality, delusional features such as incorrigibility, impossibility of content and inconsequentiality are said to become intelligible.

However, it has also been argued that positing a breakdown of ordinary intentionality misfires when trying to understand delusion specifically, as opposed to, for example, formal thought disorder, disorganization or hebephrenia.[29] Against this idea of a complete breakdown of intentionality, it has been objected that delusional people in fact display many ordinary beliefs. Furthermore, in Bellaar (2022), one of us has argued that such ordinary intentionality, as indicated by the presence of ordinary beliefs alongside delusions, is not a contingent occurrence, but in fact the condition of possibility for speaking of delusion. That is, shared modes of intentionality are required to speak of shared linguistic meaning, and shared linguistic meaning is required to attribute delusion. We can see this if we appreciate that failure to grasp conventional meanings of the terms used *excludes* people from the diagnosis of delusion, for example in children and non-native speakers. This means that the conditions that enable ordinary intentionality cannot be compromised as long as we speak of delusion, whether we name such conditions 'reality contact', 'natural self-evidence', 'frame conditions', 'the ontological framework', 'the natural attitude', 'common sense', 'the sense of reality' or 'objective certainties'. Yet this means that feelings of unreality that frequently co-occur with delusions cannot involve a loss of objective certainties either. The question thus becomes how to account for feelings of unreality without committing to compromised objective certainty. A different account of the relation between objective certainty and feelings of unreality is therefore needed.

The important difference between Wittgenstein's objective certainties and the phenomenologists' sense of reality is that, for Varga and Ratcliffe (who cites Jaspers on this), the 'sense of reality' is explicitly said to be an experiential notion: experiences of unreality take the place of a sense of reality that is considered to be ordinarily always (tacitly) experienced. Nevertheless, Ratcliffe does concede that this experience normally goes unnoticed, which warrants caution regarding the extent to which this sense of reality actually is to be considered experiential. By contrast, Wittgenstein conceives objective certainties as grammatical rather than experiential notions, manifested in ways of acting rather than in feelings of (un)certainty.[30] The inclination to explain our ability to represent (un)reality (or the loss of this ability) on the basis of feelings of (un)reality was anticipated by Wittgenstein, but he urges us to resist such an approach:

> It would be just as wrong to use an experience of meaning to explain the concept of understanding meaning as to explain reality and unreality by the experience of unreality, or the concept of the presence of a human being by the feeling of a presence. One might just as well try to explain what check is in chess by a check-feeling.[31]

It is interesting to notice that Ratcliffe compares the context of a game of chess to the context of an experienced feeling of unreality in elucidating the breakdown of intentionality that he thinks to be inherent in delusion. Wittgenstein too invokes the game of chess to analyze the enabling conditions for epistemic states or attitudes. Yet he uses it to critique the idea of invoking *feelings* of (un)reality in an analysis of (the representation of) reality: we are prompted to concede that check is not to be explained in feelings of check, and this analogy is clearly invoked to make us receptive to the idea that epistemic states or attitudes are not to be explained in terms of such feelings. Instead, we are invited to compare our epistemic practices with rule-governed games like chess, and to understand our notions like doubt, belief and knowledge as enabled by normatively guided behavior. This exegetical claim becomes even more clear in *On Certainty*, where Wittgenstein analyzes our ways of knowing or perceiving reality in terms of constitutive *norms* of knowledge – objective certainties – rather than by reference to subjective feelings of (un)reality. Following up on the argument that *delusions* cannot involve a loss of intentionality (Bellaar 2022; Klee 2004; Broome 2004, 2012; Broome & Bortolotti 2008; Radden 2011; Reimer 2011), Wittgenstein's rejection of attempts to account for intentionality in terms of feelings of (un)reality may provide a different way to coherently account for the co-occurrence of delusions and feelings of unreality.

Unreality – Wittgenstein

Wittgenstein does not share Ratcliffe's idea that an enabling condition for modes of intentionality like belief and knowledge has the form of *experienced feelings* of reality. However, this leaves open the question of how to conceive of such feelings of unreality instead. In Wittgenstein's writings, reports of such feelings receive a rather different analysis: not as a breakdown of objective certainty, but as a 'secondary sense' of the notions of 'feeling' and 'unreality'. We will outline how this notion of secondary sense applies to feelings of unreality, before turning to its relation to objective certainty and its possible application to proper delusions.

Secondary sense is a technical term used by Wittgenstein to describe a *transferred use* of language.[32] It captures the phenomenon that we sometimes spontaneously[33] use words out of their conventional context of use in a nonconventional context of use. Despite being nonconventional, this use of words is still meaningful because it *presupposes* the grasp of the conventional meaning of the constituent terms used in two ways: it is definitive of secondary sense that someone can only explain the meaning of the constituent terms he uses by reference to their conventional use, and only on the condition that he can do so can his speech-act be thought of as an instance of secondary sense.[34] The former condition distinguishes this kind of meaning from metonymic or metaphorical meaning where words may be explained as meaning something else than they usually do; the latter is required to distinguish it from nonsense. In line with the dictum that "meaning is use", Wittgenstein uses 'secondary sense' and 'secondary use' interchangeably. What is secondary is therefore the *use* or *application* of these words, and the use or application of words consists of the speech-act they are part of. Secondary sense/use therefore consists of nonconventional speech-acts: '

> the secondary use consists in applying the word with this primary use in new surroundings'.[35]

We can see the same if we consider that if, per definition, secondary sense/use is a nonconventional use, and if, per definition, the meaning of the constituent terms can only be (explained in terms of) their conventional use, then it follows that the secondary sense/use that constituent terms may have consists of the unconventional speech-act. Many examples of secondary sense are expressions that involve terms of which the conventional use can be stated by giving examples where they figure in epistemic claims, yet that now have a secondary use in the form of avowals of psychological phenomena.

Wittgenstein's best-known discussion of the notion of a 'secondary sense' of language is where he introduces the term to analyze synaesthetic expressions such as 'the vowel *e* is yellow' or when he considers expressions such as 'Wednesday is fat'.[36] In the *Philosophical Investigations*, Wittgenstein introduces this notion after his discussion of aspect-seeing. Aspect-seeing is the term he uses for our ability to see something *as* something else, for example the ambiguous picture that we can see as a duck or as a rabbit. While much secondary literature exists on aspect-perception, few commentators acknowledge that expressions of noticing aspects form a *subset* of the way language can have a secondary sense.[37] In characteristic expressions of noticing an aspect ("Now I see a duck!" "Now I see it as a wire frame"), terms or phrases conventionally used in justifiable talk of perception (of the external world) or interpretation now have a secondary use in the form of ('nonconventional') avowals of subjective experience that are not subject to justification.

Examples such as 'Wednesday is fat',[38] 'experiencing the meaning of a word',[39] recollections of dream-knowledge,[40] pretend play,[41] puzzle pictures like the 'duck-rabbit',[42] musical experience,[43] and grammatical jokes[44] may lead one to think that instances of secondary sense are restricted to creative, aesthetic or playful occasions. However, these 'frivolous' or 'unserious' occasions by no means exhaust this use of language – nor should we expect them to once we realize that the significance of this use of language resides not in the light-heartedness of playfully transgressing grammatical norms, but in the way in which such transgressions can be meaningful expansions of our mental lives. Such expansions may indeed take frivolous forms, yet Wittgenstein also includes examples such as the expressions of calculating in one's head,[45] suddenly noticing resemblances between faces,[46] and suddenly recognizing an acquaintance.[47] Most relevant to the topic of the current chapter is that Wittgenstein also mentions sinister, distressing or uncanny examples as less known instances of secondary sense: for example., some expressions of depression,[48] of déjà vu,[49] of seeing others as mere automata,[50] of feelings of unreality[51] and of hallucinations[52] – all of which are or have been associated with mental illness.[53] We will focus here on the feeling of unreality that (contemporary phenomenological) psychiatrists associate with (pre-)delusional atmosphere (Feyaerts et al., 2021b). Wittgenstein too was aware that such feelings often accompany or precede mental illness:

> The feeling of the unreality of one's surroundings. This feeling I have had once, and many have it before the onset of mental illness. Everything seems somehow not real; but not as if one saw things unclear or blurred; everything looks quite as usual. And how do I know that another has felt what I have? Because he uses the same words as I find appropriate. But why do I choose precisely the word "unreality" to express it? Surely not because of its sound. (A word of very like sound but different meaning would not do.) I choose it *because of its meaning*. But I surely *did not learn* to use the word to mean: a feeling. No; but *I learned to use it with a particular meaning and now I use it spontaneously like this*. One might say – though it may mislead – When I have learnt the word in its ordinary meaning, then I choose that meaning as a simile for my feeling. But of course what is in question here is not a simile, not a comparison of the feeling with something else.[54]

This passage makes explicit that secondary sense presupposes mastery of the ordinary conventional meaning of the terms used, that we use it spontaneously rather than that we are taught this way of expressing ourselves, and that it is a use of language that is not justifiable on the basis of comparisons or similarities, which distinguishes it from metaphor or simile. The employment of metaphor or simile can to various degrees be *justified*, depending on whether the (implicit) comparison of the source with the target is a *good* comparison. We may (dis)agree about the aptness of some metaphors, and we may ask why our interlocutor chooses this metaphor accordingly. The fact that metaphors are justifiable in this manner reveals that they may also be crafted or constructed through some form of deliberate reasoning, and that we may *choose* whether we employ literal or figurative language instead.[55] When employing secondary sensical language, by contrast, we have a spontaneous inclination to use this form of expression, rather than that we have deliberately chosen it: these words are also said to *force* themselves upon us.[56] This unjustifiability means that secondary sense is indubitable, yet it is also nonconventional – hence it functions as avowals do:

> The fact is simply that I use a word, the bearer of another technique, *as the expression of a feeling*. I use it in a new way. And wherein consists this new kind of use? Well, one thing is that I say: I have a 'feeling of unreality'--after I have, of course, learnt the use of the word "feeling" in the ordinary way. Also: the feeling is a state.[57]

Wittgenstein also questions whether there is any characteristic non-verbal behavior that warrants attributing the feeling of unreality to someone in the absence of its verbal expression:

> I know, for example, that people talk of a feeling of unreality, they say everything seems unreal to them; and now one says: everything might strike people as unreal even if they had never told anyone. *How does one know straight off that it makes sense to say "perhaps everything strikes this person as unreal, although he never speaks of it"?*[58]

The answer is that it does not straightforwardly make sense, and this is simply because the relevant experience is *constituted* by the specific *terms* spontaneously forcing themselves upon the subject. We can compare this criterial role of the inclination to say 'everything seems unreal' to the criterial role of non-verbal pain behavior. Unless there are reasons for concealing it, it does not make sense to attribute pain to someone in the absence of any characteristic inclination to display pain-behavior such as crying, grabbing one's hurt ankle and so on. Such natural pain behavior plays the same criterial role with respect to the experience of pain as the inclination to say 'everything seems unreal' plays with respect to feelings of unreality. This constitutive role of the inclination to use this verbal expression does not mean that there is no other verbal or non-verbal behavior related to this experience.[59] But the claim is that such further descriptions or behavior do not *warrant* our attribution of the feeling of unreality if it is in all sincerity denied that 'everything is somehow unreal'. These other forms of (non-)verbal behavior do not play the same logical role that the verbal expression 'everything seems unreal' plays. Someone may well reject this form of expression while still staring at the mirror, and so forth, but then it becomes questionable what warrant we have for attributing *this* feeling of unreality to him. In this way, the inclination to use this form of expression is constitutive of this experience.

In the next section, we will see that the primacy of the verbal expression thus advanced allows for a coherent combination of feelings of unreality and intact objective certainty.

Certainty and Secondary Sense

As we have seen, Wittgenstein thinks that the "feeling of unreality" is an example of a secondary sense, and it should be noted that he associates both this feeling and conflicts with objective certainties with mental illness. In line with such remarks, both have been associated with delusion or madness,[60] yet not much has been written on how these two notions meaningfully relate to each other. In this section, we will argue that secondary sensical language *presupposes* objective certainty, such that feelings of unreality thus conceived are not at odds with intact everyday certainty.

Characteristic of both secondary sense and objective certainty is that they are both indubitable, for both are not subject to justification – yet they are so for different reasons. Secondary sense is indubitable to the first person because the inclination to use *this* formulation is *constitutive* of having this experience: it could be suppressed or concealed in some circumstances, yet it makes no sense to speak of someone having these experiences without him having this inclination (ter Hark 2009a). If someone would in all openness sincerely doubt or deny this form of expression, we should not be speaking of him having this experience. This indubitability stems from this constitutively criterial role of the inclination to use this form of expression in relevant contexts.

By contrast, objective certainties are indubitable precisely because contexts of use for their articulation are lacking. They may be formulated for purposes of instruction, but whether I am objectively certain is not established by reference to my articulation of objective certainties. Rather, objective certainty is manifested precisely by *not* debating or questioning it, but by performing actions and making claims that tacitly presuppose it. As soon as it would make sense for some statement to act as a dubitable and debatable claim, it would no longer articulate an objective certainty. The indubitability of objective certainties thus consists of them crucially *not being formulated* in relevant contexts.[61]

Attributing opposing secondary sense and objective certainty is therefore logically possible because the criteria on the basis of which they are attributed do not contradict each other. Not only is this opposition quite possible, it is even the typical situation in cases of secondary sense. We can see this when we consider that *secondary* sense borrows phrases and concepts that have their ordinary use and meaning in a different language game.

These concepts like 'unreality' are *transferred* from this ordinary way of using them to their secondary use in a different language game, which we have seen to be that of avowals. This means that in order to say that someone uses words in a secondary sense, he or she must master their primary sense. And for Wittgenstein, as should be clear, the primary locus of meaning is in our normatively guided linguistic practices. Accordingly, in order for someone to sensibly use 'unreal' as part of an avowal of the feeling of unreality, he or she must be able to offer an explanation of the conventional or primary meaning or use of 'unreal'. And for many terms, including the notion of (un)reality, our conventional use lies in epistemic applications. These epistemic applications in turn are constituted by objective certainties. How does someone show she grasps such norms? Not by stating them, but by following them. As a result, a person may sensibly be said to express a feeling of unreality when she is able to *judge* things to be real and unreal in accordance with objective certainties. It follows that such a person displays a natural form of 'double-bookkeeping' (cf. Bleuler 1950) between her nonconventional secondary sense, on the one hand, and her conventional applications of the terms involved on the other.

We can illustrate the above by examining more closely expressions of feelings of unreality. We have argued that such expressions presuppose a grasp of the conventional meanings of (un)reality. We see that this condition is indeed satisfied when people who explain what they mean when they say everything seems 'unreal' resort to talk of being part of dreams, films or theater plays – all examples of events that in our epistemic practices we paradigmatically *count* as known to be unreal. By giving precisely these explanations of what she means with 'unreal', the sufferer of the unreality feeling shows herself to be quite capable of ordinary judgements of '(un)reality'. The certainty that 'I know that what happens in films, theater plays and dreams is unreal' is therefore not lost, but instead presupposed by the feeling that everything is unreal. This certainty *could* be compromised if the sufferer was no longer able to specify what she means by the notion of 'unreality' and would fail to explain herself by means of examples of what commonly counts as unreal. For example, if she elaborates what she means by giving a random selection of both real and unreal events, then we should think she lost a grasp of the notion of (un)reality. But in such a case we should be quite hesitant to identify her words as expressions of feelings of *unreality*, as opposed to a manifestation of a much more disorganized condition.

It could be objected that we cannot apply this model to delusions because people with delusions do not *tell* us they are objectively certain of not-X. But in fact some delusional people *do* tell us this.[62] Furthermore, such assurance is not even required to speak of intact certainty. In Bellaar (2022), it was argued that once we attribute delusion to someone, we already imply that she is objectively certain, such that assurance of this certainty is superfluous and the demand vacuous. But more generally, the inclination to demand assurance of objective certainty relies on confusion. When in a particular context, X functions as an objective certainty, it is meaningless to doubt whether X or not-X. But the meaningfulness of the demand for reassurance of my objective certainty that X presupposes that I can also meaningfully say that X is *not* certain to me – yet this is to confuse objective certainties for empirical propositions. While empirical claims to knowledge – and our justification thereof – are made to assure that indeed we do know, articulations of certainties are made for instructive purposes rather than to reassure that we are indeed certain. The demand for reassurance of someone's objective certainty therefore is self-defeating: as soon as I maintain that my demand for reassurance makes sense, I cannot be speaking about objective certainty, and as soon as we speak about objective certainty, demands for reassurance are meaningless. Whether a delusional person tells us she is objectively certain or not thus does not impact whether she *is* so or not. Instead, her certainty is manifested in other (non-)verbal behavior in which it is presupposed. We argued in Bellaar (2022) that the non-delusional thought and behavior that is required to meaningfully attribute delusion in the first place already manifests intact objective certainty.

Secondary Sense or Nonsense?

Now that we have seen how pre-delusional or co-delusional feelings of unreality presuppose intact objective certainty, we will explore how secondary sense is able to capture proper delusional phenomena. Thornton (2004, 2012) considers this approach to delusions, but discards it on the basis of several objections.

Thornton (2004, 2012) considers Sass's (1994) analysis of the famous schizophrenic Schreber. Thornton objects that Schreber's delusional words are not secondary sense because Schreber cannot explicate to us *what* secondary sense his words carry. This objection may be intuitive on a superficial grasp of the notion of secondary sense, but it misfires because of a misunderstanding. The notion of secondary sense/use does not entail that the meaning of words is explained in any nonconventional manner; quite the contrary: as soon as someone explains his words in a nonconventional way, we should no longer be speaking of secondary sense. Instead, the meaning of the terms used should be grasped in a conventional way – and this grasp is guaranteed by the double-bookkeeping that is inherent in delusion. The proper response to Thornton would therefore be to say that the secondary use that Schreber gives to his words consists of his delusional speech-acts, in the way a secondary use of 'fat' consists of saying 'Wednesday is fat'.

A second objection that Thornton (2004) raises is that we do not share *this* expressive use of words with delusional people. This is hardly an objection, for it is the *prerequisite* of secondary sense that it is nonconventional language, and therefore that *competent* language users *may always fail* to share the inclination to use these expressions without being *wrong* in doing so.[63] If such a use of words was conventional, we could be *wrong* in failing to see the duck in the ambiguous figure, we could be *wrong* in not thinking that '*e* is yellow', but then these would simply cease to be cases of aspect-perception or synesthesia. Hence, if understanding is modeled after shared inclinations to use these words, we may simply not understand the deluded without anyone being wrong here. And conversely, it follows that those who do share these delusional inclinations – as in folies à deux – are not *right* in their 'understanding' either.[64]

A further critical response to the current proposal could be to wonder if we have not somehow strayed too far in making room for meaningful language by including conflicts with epistemic norms in the domain of our psychological expressions. In other words: have we not now reached the point at which *any* apparent nonsense can be thought to be meaningful along the lines of secondary sense developed thus far? Can we really think of this use of language as involving actual *experiences*? Are we now committed to the idea that *anything* we say can be thought to express *an experience?* Thornton (2012) can be read as objecting in this manner, and it is a question that Wittgenstein too anticipated:

> *What* do I experience? … [D]o I merely say it? – that is, that this word meant this to me--and did *nothing* happen? It was mere words? – Not mere words; and it can also be said that something happened, which corresponded to them – but one cannot *explain* that it wasn't mere words by saying that something corresponding to them happened. For the two expressions mean the same thing.[65]

Wittgenstein stresses here in a different way the criterial role of the inclination to use this particular form of expression: because this inclination is *constitutive* of having this kind of experience, I cannot explain my use of words by offering an independent description of a state that justifies my initial formulation.

Accordingly, in order to maintain that secondary sense conveys an actual experience rather than being *mere words*, we cannot distinguish the two on the basis of (a contingent lack of) justification. This also entails that we cannot just decide to say anything at will and claim it to be secondary sense, for if we can choose the form of our expression, we should be able to justify our choice of words. But this we cannot do in cases of secondary sense, because the form of expression that we are inclined to use there is not a matter of deliberation to begin with; rather, it forces itself on us spontaneously.[66]

Of course, I can also *pretend* to have the spontaneous inclination to use this form of expression, such that I may *pretend* not to be able to justify my words. In such a case it also may be questioned whether *something happened* at all. Here, the difference with secondary sense resides in sincerity.[67] I can pretend and say 'everything seems unreal' but in doing so, I do not sincerely give in to the spontaneous inclination to use these words[68] – at best I give in to the inclination to pretend to be inclined to use these words.

We thus see that in secondary sense the expression ought to be sincere and the form of expression involuntary. This allows us to resist the objection that we have now attributed sense where there is none. Such an objection can be found in Thornton (2012), who considers a typically nonsensical combination of words such as 'milk me sugar', and maintains that since we have not given it an expressive *role* in our linguistic practices, it cannot qualify as secondary sense but should be considered nonsense instead. Thornton grants that we may suppose that he masters the conventional meanings of 'milk', 'me' and 'sugar'. Nevertheless, he maintains, a practical situation in which this particular combination of words has its use is lacking, and therefore meaning is absent – even secondary meaning. Phrases such as these can be produced at will – but this is precisely where this kind of objection misfires: the speech-acts that we can rightfully characterize in terms of secondary sense *cannot* be such that their form of expression is chosen at will. These words are not chosen for reasons that justify their use, nor are they chosen without such justification, for their spontaneity has it that they are not chosen at all. The same holds for delusions. *These* kinds of objections cannot serve as counterexamples accordingly.

We have now seen how three requirements of secondary sense are crucially met by delusional language. First, we saw that someone must master the primary meanings of the words used, and that this is constituted by objective certainties – this condition is met by the double-bookkeeping in delusion that has been demonstrated to be present on empirical grounds by Sass (1994), and on conceptual grounds elsewhere (Bellaar 2022). Second, we have seen how the delusional form of expression cannot be subject to the will in two senses: it cannot be justified, nor can the form of expression be chosen at will without sincere inclination to use these words. That delusions cannot be justified follows from their conflict with objective certainty (Bellaar 2022). Finally, that delusions are sincere speech-acts follows from the fact that pretense excludes the attribution of delusion.[69]

Conclusion: Knowledge in Delusion

Let us recapitulate: we have first considered the idea – proposed by phenomenological authors like Ratcliffe amongst others – that (pre-)delusional feelings of unreality involve a loss of objective certainty, and a breakdown of intentionality accordingly. We have rejected such a view in favor of an analysis of reports of unreality feelings in terms of secondary sense. That Schreber's delusions can be interpreted as instances of secondary sense because of his double bookkeeping has been empirically demonstrated by Sass; elsewhere (Bellaar 2022), it was argued that such double bookkeeping is conceptually inherent to delusions. We will now conclude the chapter with a proposal to see how not just Schreber's delusions, but delusions in general, are instances of secondary sense. Specifically: we will see *how* the explicit delusional use of 'I know' can be meaningful in this way.

An example of the secondary sensical employment of the notion of knowledge can be found in recollections of dreams. We may speak of knowing things in our dreams, yet outside the dream, we do not know those things we know inside the dream, or we even know the contrary. Nevertheless, we are not *wrong* in saying we knew those things in dreams: we do not wake up and realize that we merely *thought* we knew, and this shows itself in the fact that it is very odd to try or expect us to *correct* ourselves when waking up. In turn, the fact that we do not need to correct ourselves shows that we are not *incorrectly* employing the notion of knowledge when talking about knowing in our dreams. Our reports of knowledge in dreams have the form of an avowal: "In my dream I knew that I was dead" is not meaningfully challenged by counterarguments, and we can only make reference to our own state to back it up. Accordingly, we are dealing with an application of 'to know' that cannot function as a claim to knowledge, but rather functions as an avowal: 'to know' is transferred to a different language game, we are dealing with a secondary sense.[70]

Wittgenstein connects these avowals of knowledge in dreams to reports of hallucinations[71]:

> 513. [Recall] the dream phenomenon, which, in telling a dream, one describes with the words: "and I knew that …". And it also has some similarity to what is called "hallucination"
>
> (1980a)

> 965. Is a dream a hallucination? – The memory of a dream is like the memory of a hallucination, or rather: like the memory of a real experience. This means that sometimes you would like to say: "I just saw this and that", as if you really had just seen it
>
> (1982)

The use of epistemic verbs such as 'knowing' in dreams, and 'seeing' in both dreams and hallucination, shows a likeness to ordinary epistemic claims and visual reports: "I just saw this and that". But they are not reports *of* a likeness to perceptual or epistemic claims: we do not say of dreams and hallucinations that "it is as if I knew" or "it is as if I had just seen it". These are therefore transferred uses of language: secondary sense rather than simile. We thus see that dreams provide an example of transferred use of 'knowledge', whereas the expression of hallucinations provides an example of psychotic language functioning in this way. What's more, as observed by Descartes (1641/2022) and easily verified by most of us, the extraordinary or absurd character of our dreams do not prevent us to unproblematically say that we *knew* these things in our dreams. This transferred use of knowing is apparently not subject to the same restrictions as conventional uses of knowing are.[72] Therefore, if we accept that our reports of dreams are meaningful, the absurdity of the contents of delusions alone cannot prevent us from speaking of a meaningful delusional use of 'I know'. As such, we see how the meaningfulness of delusional language can be thought to be conceptually related to the meaningfulness of expressions of dreams, offering a new take on the well-known metaphor of 'psychosis as a waking dream'.[73]

In delusion too we are confronted with an application of the notion of 'knowledge' to that which is logically impossible to know by exercising our epistemic capacities.[74] And this may well be recognised by delusional people,[75] resulting in a form of double-bookkeeping:

> [P]atients carry on a kind of "double-entry bookkeeping". ... They know the real state of affairs as well as the falsified one[76]

Observations of double-bookkeeping show us that the capacity for ordinary knowledge often seems not to be compromised in delusional people.[77] But unlike Bleuler's observations and Sass's examples of Schreber's double-bookkeeping, the apparent contradiction between ordinary knowledge and delusional applications of 'knowledge' is no contingent or empirical curiosity: it has been argued on conceptual grounds that double-bookkeeping is a precondition for attributing delusion (Bellaar 2022). A situation that Freud thought 'inexplicable' without resort to the unconscious:

> The strange behaviour of patients, in being able to combine a conscious knowing with not knowing, remains inexplicable by what is called normal psychology.[78]

Wittgenstein (1998a) too grappled with the possibility of such a double-bookkeeping in the case of 'fancies', a category that contains delusion,[79] although he distinguishes the opposing forms of knowing in terms of verbalization:

> It is possible for one to live, to think, in the fancy that things are thus and so, without believing it; that is to say, when one is asked, then one knows, but if one does not have to answer the question one does not know, but acts and thinks according to another opinion.[80]

Nevertheless:

> [when a form of expression] dominates our thinking, we should like to say: "But surely it is so in some sense." Although the 'some sense' is just what matters.[81]

We can now see that the 'some sense' in which such statements can be meaningful is what Wittgenstein later called secondary sense. We are confronted with, on the one hand, a nonconventional application of 'knowledge' that is verbally manifest, and on the other hand, a conventional (grasp of) 'knowledge' that is manifest by being presupposed in other thought and action. We have seen that this grasp of conventional meaning is an enabling condition for the use of words in a secondary sense – and we have seen that this condition is met by the delusional use of the notion of knowledge (Bellaar 2022). Moreover, sincerity and involuntariness allow us to distinguish this use of 'I know' from *mere words* or nonsense. Secondary sense therefore offers a conceptual tool that allows us to see *how* the delusional 'I know' can be meaningful while unable to report conventional knowledge. Delusional statements can thus be understood as avowals of knowledge, rather than claims to knowledge, normative statements of (what counts as) knowledge, or even nonsensical uses of 'knowledge'.

With delusional statements of knowledge rendered intelligible in a first-person use, we may now wonder whether a third-person use is coherent too. We maintain it is. To say of someone that he *knows* to be Christ is in every way *at least* as telling of his delusion as to say of him that he merely mistakenly thinks to know to be Christ – yet it does justice to both the words of the patient and their specific delusional irrationality. And we do not risk confusion, or perhaps even committing *ourselves* to delusional talk. To say of someone else that 'he knows to be Christ' need not commit us to saying that *we* (can) know him to be, just as saying 'she hears voices' does not commit us to saying that we (can) hear those voices ourselves, or when we say of someone 'he knew in his dream to be president' does not commit us to saying that we knew or (can) know him to be. The third-person ascriptions of delusions in this way are not delusional themselves.

After all, we have already seen that delusional statements have the form of an avowal (Bellaar 2022), and when we speak in this way about *someone else* we are not making an avowal, for our attribution is both dubitable and predicated by reference to someone else rather than to ourselves. Hence, we would not be avowing a delusion in saying so, and therefore we cannot be said to be delusional ourselves. Instead, we are attributing to someone else a *state* that is criterially constituted by *his* avowal 'I know that …'.[82]

To conclude: in the foregoing, we have not presented a 'radically empathic' understanding of someone's situation that offers *better* words to articulate it than the person himself does (e.g., Ratcliffe 2012). The delusional 'I know' is not an indirect or convoluted way to say something that does *not* display the specific delusional irrationality. As soon as we can readily formulate 'the real meaning' of delusional statements in terms that do not display this delusional irrationality, we should no longer be speaking of delusion. Rather, here we have come to a form of understanding of the very words delusional persons already use themselves.[83] We have come to see *how* someone can meaningfully say 'I know' here rather than *why*. To ask *why* delusional people say what they say is to already presuppose that delusions are subject to justification – but this is already to ask the wrong question, for justification is precisely what the specific delusional irrationality precludes.[84] Hence, delusions cannot be sensibly conceptualized as beliefs or *claims* to knowledge – for such are subject to justification. Since *avowals of knowledge* are not subject to justification, delusional conflicts with objective certainties logically can take such a form instead. We have now seen how the notion of secondary sense allows us to understand how delusional language can indeed be meaningful in this way. Delusions are thus meaningfully said to be a form of knowledge, yet their specific irrationality means that they logically cannot *function* as knowledge. Hence, delusions are *pathological knowledge*, or – as Jaspers says – *a morbid manifestation of knowledge*.[85] This analysis allows us to both acknowledge the words of the patient, while regarding them as delusional nonetheless. We now have the conceptual resources to confidently say that we believe the patient knows herself to be Christ, yet simultaneously that *we* cannot know her to be so.[86] And this is a characterization of delusion that may be shared both by patient and therapist; it provides a foothold for *agreement* rather than antagonism.[87]

Notes

1 Spitzer 1990.
2 APA 1994, 2013.
3 See Feyaerts et al. 2021a.

4 Bortolotti 2010, Bellaar 2022.
5 Wittgenstein 1974; Eilan 2001; Klee 2004; Sass 2004; Broome 2004; Gipps & Fulford 2004; Moyal-Sharrock 2004; Hamilton 2007; Gipps & Rhodes 2008, 2011; Cardella 2020; Frèrejouan 2021.
6 Bellaar 2022.
7 Thornton 2008; Gipps & Rhodes 2008, 2011; Fuchs 2015, 2020; van Duppen 2017; Van Duppen & Sips 2018; Boncompagni 2018; Ariso 2019; Jeppsson 2021.
8 Bellaar 2022.
9 Klee 2004; Broome 2004, 2012; Broome & Bortolotti 2008; Radden 2011; Reimer 2011.
10 Bellaar 2022.
11 Recently, Louis (2021) argued this on linguistic grounds, whereas Spitzer (1990) and Henriksen & Parnas (2014) propose the same as a way of accounting for well-known features of delusion such as certainty, incorrigibility and self-referentiality.
12 Ratcliffe 2008, 2015, 2017, Varga 2012a, 2012b.
13 That delusions are experiences was proposed already by Jaspers (1913/1963) and Conrad (Mishara 2010) on phenomenological grounds, and that delusional language has the form of expressions or avowals rather than of epistemic statements can arguably be derived from this.
14 Ratcliffe (2013), p. 232.
15 Gipps (2010).
16 Cermolacce et al. (2010).
17 Parnas & Henriksen (2013), Sass & Pienkos (2013), Parnas (2014), Sass & Byrom (2015).
18 Bovet & Parnas (1993), Stanghellini (2000, 2001, 2007, 2008), Parnas & Sass (2001), Thoma & Fuchs (2017) and Fuchs (2015, 2020).
19 Blankenburg & Mishara (2001), Boncompagni (2018).
20 Sass & Pienkos (2013), Henriksen & Parnas (2014), Sass & Byrom (2015), Bizzarri (2018).
21 Henriksen & Parnas (2014), Sass & Byrom (2015).
22 Ratcliffe (2008, 2015, 2017).
23 Varga (2012a, 2012b).
24 Ratcliffe (2017, p. 154).
25 Ratcliffe (2008, p. 171).
26 Ratcliffe (2015, p. 102).
27 Varga (2012b).
28 Ratcliffe (2013, p. 232).
29 Broome 2004, 2012; Broome & Bortolotti 2008, and conceded in Varga 2012b, see *Certainty and Delusion*.
30 Wittgenstein (1974, 494, 524).
31 Wittgenstein (1980a, 155).
32 Ter Hark (2006).
33 We are not *taught* this way of expressing ourselves as replacements for more primitively expressed states.
34 Ter Hark (2006).
35 Wittgenstein (1982: 797), see also Wittgenstein (1958, p. 216), Wittgenstein (1982: 61, 77) and Wittgenstein (1980a: 125–126).
36 Wittgenstein (1958, p. 216).

37 Though argued for by ter Hark (2009a, 2011), and observed by Agam-Segal (2012, 2014). See, e.g., Wittgenstein (1980a: 12, 20, 412, 864, 1025), Wittgenstein (1980b: 370–371, 378), and Wittgenstein (1982: 176, 179, 447, 450) where expressions of noticing aspects are described as nonconventional uses of what conventionally functions as perceptual/epistemic language, i.e., where expressions of noticing aspects are instances of secondary sense. At other occasions too, cases of secondary sense and aspects are related: Wittgenstein (1980a: 16, 1064), Wittgenstein (1980b: 375, 537, 631) Wittgenstein (1982: 175), Wittgenstein (1958, p. 202, p. 210, p. 214).
38 Wittgenstein (1958, p. 216).
39 Wittgenstein (1980a, 1060–1062).
40 Wittgenstein (1980b, 574; 1982, 57).
41 Wittgenstein (1982, 800).
42 Wittgenstein (1958, p. 194).
43 Wittgenstein (1958, 208).
44 Wittgenstein (1980a, 77).
45 Wittgenstein (1958, p. 216).
46 Wittgenstein (1980a, 692).
47 Wittgenstein (1958, p. 197).
48 Wittgenstein (1980a, 133).
49 Wittgenstein (1980a, 120, 336).
50 Wittgenstein (1958, 420).
51 Wittgenstein (1980a, 125).
52 Wittgenstein (1982, 985, 1980a, 513).
53 Wittgenstein (1982: 69, 73; 1980a, 355, 965) explicitly considers instances of secondary sense to be forms of *pathology*, *mirage*, *fancy* or *madness*.
54 Wittgenstein (1980a, 125).
55 That we can choose whether we use metaphorical language also implies Wittgenstein's dogma that what can be put figuratively can also be put literally.
56 Wittgenstein (1958, p. 197, p. 204, p. 215), Moyal-Sharrock (2000), ter Hark (2010).
57 Wittgenstein (1980a, 126).
58 Wittgenstein (1980a, 156).
59 Some people may be able to take a descriptive attitude towards the experience and employ metaphors or comparisons to further elaborate on it – some may be able to do this much more elaborate than others. Some non-verbal behavior that may be associated with the feeling may be discerned too: staring in the mirror, stamping on the floor, etc.
60 Thornton 2004, 2012; Gipps & Rhodes 2008; Gipps 2012, Frérejouan 2021, Wittgenstein 1980a: 965.
61 It should be stressed that the question of (un)altered certainties in delusional people may seem an utterly theoretical matter. There is a lot of truth in this, because typically, we do not even have much use for *attributing* objective certainties to other people, precisely because they are presupposed in a language game that mature speakers are competent in. Objective certainties are unquestionable and this can be put in two ways: we do not question that they are certain, yet also, we do not question whether they are certain *to someone*. In philosophical contexts, we may attribute these certainties to someone on the basis of him performing non-verbal actions, or verbal actions that presuppose it, rather than on the basis of someone's formulation of them.

62 Sass (2014, p. 139; David 1990 p. 804). See also the qualitative study on delusional experience by Feyaerts et al. (2021b) – in particular the section on 'double bookkeeping'.
63 Wittgenstein (1980b, 548), Baz (2020, p. 6).
64 We thus see in folie à deux that the unjustifiable meaning of delusions is mirrored by an unjustifiable form of understanding. Wittgenstein calls such understanding 'intransitive' or 'intuitive', as opposed to 'transitive' or 'discursive', where linguistic understanding consists in being able to replace or to paraphrase. (Pichler 2016, p. 53–54; Wittgenstein 1958, 531, 610).
65 Wittgenstein (1980a, 119).
66 In secondary sense, the form of expression cannot be chosen at will. This includes cases of aspect-seeing: I cannot just see anything as anything at will. However, in aspect-seeing, *whether* I see an aspect that is suggested to me is voluntary, for someone may ask or invite me to try to see, e.g., the ambiguous figure as a duck. It is important to notice that upon such an invitation, the form of expression is not chosen by me but suggested to me by the interlocutor, who in turn is subject to the criteria of spontaneity and sincerity.
67 Wittgenstein (1980a, 1003).
68 Moyal-Sharrock (2000).
69 The two conditions for secondary sense allow us to distinguish between delusion, disorganized language and made-up nonsense such as Thornton's 'milk me sugar'. Disorganization is characterized by a lack of a grasp of ordinary meanings – a loss of objective certainties, yet may not be considered a willful *choice* of words. Made-up nonsense is advanced by people who may grasp primary meanings and adhere to objective certainties, yet is voluntary with respect to its content.
70 Wittgenstein 1980b, 574; 1982, 57.
71 See also Marchesin (2021).
72 And we can see why: claims to knowledge require the possibility of justification. Since conflicts with objective certainties cannot sensibly be thought to be justified, they cannot sensibly be thought to be *claims* to knowledge. Since avowals are not subject to justification to begin with, in making delusional avowals I am not committed to (the possibility of) justification. Conflicts with objective certainties therefore are able to take the form of avowals.
73 As traceable to Kant (1798/2006, p. 114), and recently Ritunnano & Bortolotti (2022), Sass & Pienkos (2013), Sass (2014). While reports of both dreams and delusions may be secondary uses of 'knowing', they are not to be equated. One cannot be attributed delusion solely on the basis of reports of dreams, and one cannot be said to have some dream solely on the basis of reports of delusion. Instead, the difference is already stated in the 'psychosis as a waking dream' comparison: it resides in the conceptual fact that expressions of dreams are retrospective on a sleep state, whereas expressions of delusions pertain to waking states.
74 We cannot attempt to obtain a delusion.
75 Feyaerts *et al.* 2021b.
76 Bleuler 1950, p. 56.
77 Klee 2004; Broome 2004, 2012; Broome & Bortolotti 2008; Radden 2011; Reimer 2011; Sass 1994, 2014.
78 Freud 1913, p. 142 as cited in David 1990.
79 Ter Hark (1990) argues that Wittgenstein's use of '*einbildung*', which is translated as 'fancy', covers the notion of delusion.

80 Wittgenstein (1998a) appendix II 12 p.115.
81 Wittgenstein (1998a) appendix II 13 p.116.
82 To say of the hallucinating psychotic that 'he hears voices' is just to say 'he says he hears voices, and he is sincere', and the same treatment can be given to reports of knowledge in dreams: 'in his dream, he knew to be Christ' and so 'in his delusion, he knew to be Christ' is no more than 'he says he knows to be Christ, and he is sincere'. We can even do away with the qualification 'in his delusion', for to say one knows to be Christ while awake is already delusional, such that the qualification 'in his delusion' is superfluous. Some may object that delusional people do not defend their sincerity when their delusion is challenged. This is a confused objection, for while delusional people may indeed not respond like this when their professed knowledge is challenged, they most likely will respond like this when they are charged with insincerity.
83 It is the words *the patients themselves* use that warrant the attribution of delusion: we do not need to interpret patients' words before we can come to realize they are delusional. If we want to understand *delusions*, we therefore want to see how the words used by patients themselves are intelligible. If we have a problem understanding those words, and 'solve' this by imposing upon such words a translation into words we *do* understand, it is questionable whether we now understand the deluded or rather our own fantasy of them.
84 A resort can of course be to maintain that delusional language is metaphorical (e.g., Cermolacce et al. 2010), yet if its real meaning is some state(ment) that *can* be justified, it simply ceases to be a delusion.
85 Jaspers (1963, p. 99, 103, 105, 108).
86 It could of course be objected that such a conclusion may seem awry in a conceptual analysis of delusion: many people simply do not speak of delusions as a form of knowledge, and feel uneasy to use the notion of knowledge to talk about delusions. This is true, but an important majority of people talking about delusions do use the notion of knowledge to talk about them, and would feel quite uneasy not to. This group of course consists of delusional people themselves. What we have shown here is that there is no contradiction between endorsing such a use of 'knowledge' here and our own assessment of these people as delusional, and that no opposition between the two need be perceived.
87 To conclude, we may respond to possible objections to the current proposal by means of contraposition. If someone were to say 'all right, this is an intelligible possibility but it still does not capture *delusion*', then our response could be: if you agree that this transferred use of the notion of knowledge is a coherent possibility, what kind of speech-act would this then be *if not* delusional?' If the possibility of qualifying language as delusional implies that we cannot analyze it as we have done, then by contraposition this holds as well: if we can analyze language in the way we have done, then we cannot qualify it as delusional. But what kind of speech-act would such a use of the notion of knowledge be instead?.

References

Agam-Segal, R. (2012). "How to investigate the grammar of aspect-perception: A question in Wittgensteinian method", *Essays Philosophy*, 13, pp. 85–105.
Agam-Segal, R. (2014). "When language gives out: Conceptualization and aspect-seeing as a form of judgment", *Metaphilosophy*, 45(1), pp. 41–68.

American Psychiatric Association (APA) (1994), *Diagnostic and Statistical Manual for Mental Disorders*, 4th edition, American Psychiatric Association, Washington, DC.

American Psychiatric Association (APA) (2013), *Diagnostic and Statistical Manual for Mental Disorders*, 5th edition, American Psychiatric Publishing, Arlington.

Ariso, J. (2019). "Delusion formation through uncertainty and possibility-blindness", *Logos Anales del Seminario de Metafísica*, 52, pp. 29–50, https://doi.org/10.5209/asem.65851

Baz, A. (2020). *Wittgenstein on Aspect Perception*, Cambridge University Press, Cambridge.

Bellaar, R. (2022). "Certainty and delusion", *Philosophical Psychology*, https://doi.org/10.1080/09515089.2022.2125372

Bizzarri, V. (2018). "Schizophrenia and Common Sense: A Phenomenological Perspective", in Hipolito, I. et al (eds.), *Schizophrenia and Common Sense*, Springer, Cham, pp. 39–53.

Blankenburg, W. & Mishara, A. (2001). "First steps toward a psychopathology of 'common sense'", *Philosophy, Psychiatry, and Psychology*, 8(4), pp. 303–315, https://doi.org/10.1353/ppp.2002.0014

Bleuler, E. (1950). *Dementia Preacox or the Group of Schizophrenias.* Translated by J. Zinkin, International Universities Press, New York.

Boncompagni, A. (2018). "Common Sense, Philosophy, and Mental Disturbance: A Wittgensteinian Outlook", in Hipólito, I., Gonçalves, J., & Pereira, J. (eds.), *Schizophrenia and Common Sense. Studies in Brain and Mind*, vol. 12. Springer, Cham. https://doi.org/10.1007/978-3-319-73993-9_14

Bortolotti, L. (2010). *Delusions and other Irrational Beliefs*, Oxford University Press, Oxford.

Bortolotti, L. (2020). "Doctors without 'disorders'", *Aristotelian Society Supplementary*, 94(1), 163–184, https://doi.org/10.1093/ARISUP/AKAA006

Bovet, P. & Parnas, J. (1993). "Schizophrenic delusions: A phenomenological approach", *Schizophrenia Bulletin*, 19(3), pp. 579–597.

Brenner, W. (2005). "Wittgenstein's Kantian Solution", in Brenner, W. & Moyal-Sharrock, D. (eds.), *Readings of Wittgenstein's on Certainty*, Palgrave MacMillan, Houndmills, pp. 122–141.

Broome, M. (2004). "The rationality of psychosis and understanding the deluded", *Philosophy, Psychiatry, and Psychology*, 11 (1), pp. 35–41, https://doi.org/10.1353/ppp.2004.0035

Broome, M. (2012). "Reality, realness, and the natural attitude", *Philosophy, Psychiatry and Psychology*, 19 (2), pp. 115–118, https://doi.org/10.1353/ppp.2012.0022

Broome, M. & Bortolotti, L. (2008). "Delusional beliefs and reason giving", *Philosophical Psychology*, 21 (6), pp. 821–841 https://doi.org/10.1080/09515080802516212

Cardella, V. (2020). "Rationality in mental disorders: Too little or too much?", *European Journal of Analytic Philosophy*, 16(2), pp. 13–36, https://doi.org/10.31820/ejap.16.2.1

Cermolacce, M., et al. (2010). "What is Bizarre in Bizarre delusions? A critical review", *Schizophrenia Bulletin*, 36(4), pp. 667–697, https://doi.org/10.1093/schbul/sbq001

David, A. S. (1990). "Insight and psychosis", *BJPsych*, 156, pp. 798–808.

Descartes, R. (1641/2022). *Meditations on First Philosophy*. Translated by J. Veitch, Ryerson University, Toronto.

van Duppen, Z. (2017). "The intersubjective dimension of schizophrenia", *Philosophy, Psychiatry and Psychology*, 24(4), pp. 399–418, https://doi.org/10.1353/ppp.2017.0058

van Duppen, Z. & Sips, R. (2018). "Understanding the blind spots of psychosis: A wittgensteinian and first-person approach", *Psychopathology*, 51, pp. 276–284, https://doi.org/10.1159/000490257

Eilan, N. (2001). "Meaning, truth, and the self: Commentary on Campbell and Parnass and sass", *Philosophy, Psychiatry, and Psychology*, 8(2–3), pp. 121–132, https://doi.org/10.1353/ppp.2001.0008

Feyaerts, J., et al. (2021a). "Delusions beyond beliefs: A critical overview of diagnostic, aetiological, and therapeutic schizophrenia research from a clinical-phenomenological perspective", *The Lancet Psychiatry*, 8(3), pp. 237–249, https://doi.org/10.1016/S2215-0366(20)30460-0

Feyaerts, J., et al. (2021b). "Uncovering the realities of delusional experience in schizophrenia: A qualitative phenomenological study in Belgium", *The Lancet Psychiatry*, 8(9), pp. 784–796, https://doi.org/10.1016/S2215-0366(21)00196-6

Frèrejouan, M. (2021). "The Myth of Irrationality: A Wittgensteinian Approach to Delusions and to the Principle of Charity", in Amblard, M., Musiol, M., & Rebuschi, M. (eds.), *(In)coherence of Discourse*, Springer, Cham, pp. 131–152, https://doi.org/10.1007/978-3-030-71434-5

Freud, S. (1913). "On Beginning the Treatment (Further Recommendations on the Technique of Psychoanalysis I)", *Standard Edition* (1958), vol. 12. Hogarth Press, London, pp. 123–144.

Fuchs, T. (2015). "Pathologies of intersubjectivity in Autism and Schizophrenia", *Journal of Consciousness Studies*, 22(1–2), pp. 191–214.

Fuchs, T. (2020). "Delusion, reality, and intersubjectivity: A phenomenological and enactive analysis", *Philosophy, Psychiatry & Psychology*, 27(1), pp. 61–79, https://doi.org/10.1353/ppp.2020.0009

Gipps, R. (2010). "The intelligibility of delusion", *Current Opinions in Psychiatry*, 23, pp. 556–560.

Gipps, R. G. T. (2012). "The indefinability and unintelligibility of delusion", *Philosophy, Psychiatry, & Psychology*. 19(2), pp. 91–95. https://www.muse.jhu.edu/article/484343

Gipps, R. & Fulford, K. (2004). "Understanding the clinical concept of delusion: From an estranged to an engaged epistemology", *International Review of Psychiatry*, 16, pp. 1–11, https://doi.org/10.1080/09540260400003966

Gipps, R., & Rhodes, J. (2008). "Delusions, certainty, and the background", *Philosophy, Psychiatry, and Psychology*, 15(4), pp. 295–310, https://doi.org/10.1353/ppp.0.0202

Gipps, R. & Rhodes, J. (2011). "Delusions and the non-epistemic foundations of belief", *Philosophy, Psychiatry, and Psychology*, 18(1), pp. 89–97, https://doi.org/10.1353/ppp.2011.0002

Hamilton, A. (2007). "Against the Belief Model of Delusion", in Chung, M., Fulford, K., & Graham, G. (eds.), *Reconceiving Schizophrenia*, Oxford University Press, Oxford, pp. 217–234

ter Hark, M. (1990). *Beyond the Inner and the Outer*, Kluwer Academic Publishers, Dordrecht.

ter Hark, M. (2006). "Wittgenstein, pretend play and the transferred use of language", *Journal of the Theory of Social Behavior*, 36(3), pp. 299–319, https://doi.org/10.1111/j.1468-5914.2006.00308.x

ter Hark, M. (2009a). "Coloured vowels: Wittgenstein on Synaesthesia and secondary meaning", *Philosophia*, 37, pp. 589–604 https://doi.org/10.1007/s11406-009-9194-4

ter Hark, M. (2009b). "Wittgenstein, the Secondary Use of Words, and Child Psychology", in Levy, D. & Zamuner, E. (eds.), *Wittgenstein's Enduring Arguments*, Routledge, New York.

ter Hark, M. (2010). "Experience of meaning, secondary use and aesthetics", *Philosophical Investigations*, 33(2), pp. 142–158, https://doi.org/10.1111/j.1467-9205.2010.01405.x

ter Hark, M. (2011). "Wittgenstein on the Experience of Meaning and Secondary Use", in Kuusela, O., & McGinn, M. (eds.), *The Oxford Handbook of Wittgenstein*, Oxford University Press, Oxford.

Henriksen, M. (2013). "On inconprehensibility in schizophrenia", *Phenomenology and the Cognitive Sciences*, 12, pp. 105–129, https://doi.org/10.1007/s11097-010-9194-7

Henriksen, M. & Parnas, J. (2014). "Self-disorders and schizophrenia: A phenomenological reappraisal of poor insight and noncompliance", *Schizophrenia Bulletin*, 40(3), pp. 542–547, https://doi.org/10.1093/schbul/sbt087

Hinzen, W., et al. (2016). "Can delusions be understood linguistically?" *Cognitive Neuropsychiatry*, 21(4), pp. 281–299, https://doi.org/10.1080/13546805.2016.1190703

Jaspers, K. (1963). *General Psychopathology*. Translated by J. Hoenig, G. E. M. Anscombe, & M. W. Hamilton, Manchester University Press, Manchester.

Jeppsson, S. (2021). "Psychosis and intelligibility", *Philosophy, Psychiatry and Psychology*, 28(3), pp. 233–249, https://doi.org/10.1353/ppp.2021.0036

Kant, I. (1798/2006). *Anthropology from a Pragmatic Point of View*. Translated and edited by R. Louden, Cambridge University Press, Cambridge.

Klee, R. (2004). "Why some delusions are necessarily inexplicable beliefs", *Philosophy, Psychiatry, and Psychology*, 11(1), pp. 25–34, https://doi.org/10.1353/ppp.2004.0044

Louis, F. (2021). "Incoherent Discourse in Schizophrenia: An Anthropological Approach to the Mind", in Amblard, M., Musiol, M., & Rebuschi, M., (eds.), *(In)coherence of Discourse*, Springer, Cham, pp. 153–170, https://doi.org/10.1007/978-3-030-71434-5_8

Marchesin, M. (2021). "Wittgenstein's Late Account of Meaning a Non-Normative Point of View", Doctoral Thesis, University of East Anglia.

Mishara, A. (2010). "Klaus Conrad (1905–1961): Delusional mood, psychosis, and beginning 219 Schizophrenia", *Schizophrenia Bulletin*, 36(1), pp. 9–13, https://doi.org/10.1093/schbul/sbp144

Moyal-Sharrock, D. (2000). "Words as deeds: Wittgenstein's 'spontaneous utterances' and the dissolution of the explanatory gap", *Philosophical Psychology*, 13(3), pp. 355–372 https://doi.org/10.1080/09515080050128169

Moyal-Sharrock, D. (2004). *Understanding Wittgenstein's on Certainty*, Palgrave Macmillan, Houndmills.

Parnas, J. & Sass, L. (2001). "Self, solipsism, and schizophrenic delusions", *Philosophy, Psychiatry, and Psychology*. 8(2/3), pp. 101–120, https://doi.org/10.1353/ppp.2001.0014

Parnas, J. & Henriksen, M. (2013). "Subjectivity and schizophrenia: Another look at incomprehensibility and treatment nonadherence", *Psychopathology*, 46(5), pp. 320–329, https://doi.org/10.1159/000351837

Parnas, J. (2013). "On Psychosis: Karl Jaspers and Beyond", in Stanghellini, G. & Fuchs, T. (eds.), *One Century of Karl Jaspers' General Psychopathology*, Oxford University Press, Oxford, pp. 208–228.

Parnas, J. (2014). "Philosophical and Phenomenological Perspectives on Psychosis", in Waters, F. & Stephane, M. (eds.), *The Assessment of Psychosis*, Routledge, New York, pp. 17–43.

Pichler, G. Eugene. (2016). *The Transsexual Delusion*. Lulu.com.

Poupart, F., et al. (2021). "Acting on delusion and delusional inconsequentiality: A review", *Comprehensive Psychiatry*, 106, 152230, https://doi.org/10.1016/j.comppsych.2021.152230

Radden, J. (2011). *On Delusion*, Routledge, New York.

Ratcliffe, M. (2008). *Feelings of Being: Phenomenology, psychiatry and the sense of reality*, Oxford University Press, Oxford.

Ratcliffe, M. (2012). "Phenomenology as a form of empathy", *Inquiry*, 55(5), pp. 473–495, http://doi.org/10.1080/0020174X.2012.716196

Ratcliffe, M. (2013). "Delusional Atmosphere and the Sense of Unreality", in Stanghellini, G., & Fuchs, T. (eds.), *One Century of Karl Jaspers' General Psychopathology*, Oxford University Press, Oxford.

Ratcliffe, M. (2015). "How is Perceptual Experience Possible? The Phenomenology of Presence and the Nature of Hallucination", in Breyer, Doyon M. (ed.), *Normativity in Perception. New Directions in Philosophy and Cognitive Science*, Palgrave Macmillan, London.

Ratcliffe, M. (2017). *Real Hallucinations: Psychiatric Illness, Intentionality, and the Interpersonal World*, MIT Press, Cambridge MA.

Read, R. (2001). "On approaching schizophrenia through Wittgenstein", *Philosophical Psychology*, 14(4), pp. 449–475, https://doi.org/10.1080/09515080120088111

Read, R. (2003). "Literature as philosophy of psychopathology: William Faulkner as Wittgenstein", *Philosophy, Psychiatry, & Psychology*, 10(2), pp. 115–124, https://doi.org/10.1353/ppp.2003.0099

Reimer, M. (2011). "A Davidsonian perspective on psychiatric delusions", *Philosophical Psychology*, 24(5), pp. 659–677, https://doi.org/10.1080/09515089.2011.562642

Ritunnano, R., & Bortolotti, L. (2022). "Do delusions have and give meaning?" *Phenomenology and the Cognitive Sciences*, 21, pp. 949–968.
Sass, L. (1994). *The Paradoxes of Delusion*, Cornell University Press, Ithaca.
Sass, L. (2003). "Incomprehensibility and understanding: On interpretation of Severe Mental Illness", *Philosophy, Psychiatry, & Psychology*, 10(2), pp. 125–132, https://doi.org/10.1353/ppp.2003.0101
Sass, L. (2004). "Some reflections on the (analytic) philosophical approach to delusion", *Philosophy, Psychiatry, & Psychology*, 11(1), pp. 71–80, https://doi.org/10.1353/ppp.2004.0047
Sass, L. (2014). "Delusion and Double-Bookkeeping", in *Karl Jaspers' Philosophy & Psychopathology* (eds.), Fuchs, T., Breyer, T., & Mundt, C., Springer, New York, pp. 125–147.
Sass, L. & Pienkos, E. (2013). "Delusions: The Phenomenological Approach", in Fulford, W., Davies, M., Graham, G., Sadler, J., & Stanghellini, G. (eds.), *Oxford Handbook of Philosophy of Psychiatry*, Oxford University Press, Oxford, pp. 632–657.
Sass, L. & Byrom, G. (2015). "Phenomenological and neurocognitive perspectives on delusions: A critical overview", *World Psychiatry*, 14, pp. 164–173.
Spitzer, M. (1990). "On defining delusions", *Comprehensive Psychiatry*, 31(5), pp. 377–397, https://doi.org/10.1016/0010-440X(90)90023-L
Stanghellini, G. (2000). "Vulnerability to schizophrenia and lack of common sense", *Schizophrenia Bulletin*, 26(4), pp. 775–787, https://doi.org/10.1093/oxfordjournals.schbul.a033493
Stanghellini, G. (2001). "Psychopathology of common sense", *Philosophy, Psychiatry, and Psychology*, 8(2/3), pp. 201–218, https://doi.org/10.1353/ppp.2001.0018
Stanghellini, G. (2007). "Schizophrenia and the 6th Sense", in Chung, M., Filford, K., & Graham, G. (eds.), *Reconceiving Schizophrenia*, Oxford University Press, Oxford, pp. 129–149.
Stanghellini, G. (2008). "Schizophrenic delusions, embodiment and the background", *Philosophy, Psychiatry, and Psychology*, 15(4), pp. 311–314, https://doi.org/10.1353/ppp.0.0204
Tamelini, G. & Messas, M. (2016). "On the phenomenology of delusion: The revelation of its aprioristic structures and the consequences for clinical practice", *Psicopatologia Fenomenológica Contemporânea*, 5(1), pp. 1–21.
Thoma, S. & Fuchs, T. (2017). "A Phenomenology of Sensus Communis – Outline of a Phenomenological Approach to Social Psychiatry", in Englander, M. (ed.), *Phenomenology and the Social Context of Psychiatry. Social Relations, Psychopathology, and Husserl's Philosophy*, Bloomsbury Publishing, London, pp. 137–160.
Thornton, T. (2004). "Wittgenstein and the limits of empathic understanding in psychopathology", *International Review of Psychiatry*, 16(3), pp. 216–224, https://doi.org/10.1080/09540260400003933
Thornton, T. (2008). "Why the idea of framework propositions cannot contribute to an understanding of delusions", *Phenomenology and the Cognitive Sciences*, 7, pp. 159–175, https://doi.org/10.1007/s11097-007-9079-6

Thornton, T. (2012). "Delusional atmosphere, the everyday uncanny, and the limits of secondary sense", *Emotion Review*, 4(2), pp. 92–196, https://doi.org/10.1177%2F1754073911430137

Varga, S. (2012a). "Depersonalization and the sense of realness", *Philosophy, Psychiatry and Psychology*, 19(2), pp. 103–113.

Varga, S. (2012b). "Realness, expression, and the role of others", *Philosophy, Psychiatry and Psychology*, 19(2), pp. 123–126.

Wittgenstein, L. (1958). *Philosophical Investigations.* Translated by G. E. M. Anscombe, 2nd edition, Basil Blackwell, Oxford.

Wittgenstein, L. (1974). *On Certainty.* Edited by Anscombe, G. E. M. & von Wright, G. H., Basil Blackwell, Oxford.

Wittgenstein, L. (1980a). *Remarks on the Philosophy of Psychology*, volume 1. Edited by von Wright, G. H., & Anscombe, G. E. M., Basil Blackwell, Oxford.

Wittgenstein, L. (1980b). *Remarks on the Philosophy of Psychology*, volume 2. Edited by von Wright, G. H., & Nyman, H., Basil Blackwell, Oxford.

Wittgenstein, L. (1982). *Last Writings on the Philosophy of Psychology*, vol. 1. Edited by von Wright, G. H., & Nyman, H., Basil Blackwell, Oxford.

Wittgenstein, L. (1998a). *Remarks on the Foundations of Mathematics.* Edited by von Wright, G. H., Rhees, R., & Anscombe, G. E. M., Basil Blackwell, Oxford.

Wittgenstein, L. (1998b). *The Blue and Brown Books*, Blackwell, Oxford.

Wittgenstein, L. (1998c). *Zettel.* Edited by von Wright, G. H., Rhees, R., & Anscombe, G. E. M., Basil Blackwell, Oxford.

6 Delusional Realities, World-Traveling and Transitional Objects

Ashleigh Morales and Shaun Gallagher

Introduction

> To say simply that a delusion is a mistaken idea which is firmly held by the patient and which cannot be corrected gives only a superficial and incorrect answer to the problem ... [A]ll experience of reality ... has a root in the practice of living. ... Delusion proper ... implies a transformation in our total awareness of reality.
>
> (Jaspers 1913/1963, pp. 93–94)

According to the DSM-IV, a delusion is "a false belief based on incorrect inference about external reality" (APA, 2000, 2013: 819). The DSM-5 updates the definition: delusions are "fixed beliefs that are not amenable to change in light of conflicting evidence (ibid.). In both the philosophical and psychological literature, one also finds delusion characterized in terms of beliefs, or sometimes special sorts of beliefs such as framework beliefs, or what are sometimes called, following Wittgenstein, 'hinge propositions' (Campbell 2001). Naomi Eilan (2000, pp. 108–109) explains this view as follows.

> Our framework beliefs are those fundamental beliefs we do not question, and which globally constrain our inferences and our interpretation of our experiences. ... The suggestion is that primary paranoid beliefs ... should be treated as constraining one's reasoning and interpretation of one's experience in an analogous manner. They are resistant to counter-evidence because of their fundamental framing role.

Delusions on this view function as framework propositions and can remain relatively circumscribed and heterogeneous. Within their particular area of relevance, they can govern a variety of factual beliefs. The delusional subject may hold perplexing and paradoxical beliefs with regard to some areas of his life, but be relatively rational in others. Consistent with the

DOI: 10.4324/9781003288992-9

DSM's characterization of delusions, such framework beliefs remain "firmly sustained despite what almost everyone else believes and despite what constitutes incontrovertible and obvious proof or evidence to the contrary."

To consider a delusion to be merely a belief, or even a special type of framework belief, however, is, as Jaspers suggested, to abstract it from something much richer – something that the delusional subject experiences and lives through. In order to capture this richer experience, in this chapter we propose an alternative characterization of delusion, making use of both phenomenological and cultural studies, specifically concepts drawn from the work of Alfred Schutz on multiple realities, and Maria Lugones on world-traveling.

Multiple Realities and World-Traveling

On phenomenologically inspired enactive accounts of human action and experience, an agent is not first and foremost an intellectual creature who perceives the world objectively or abstractly, and then formulates her beliefs, and acts accordingly upon those beliefs. Rather, the experiencing subject is first and foremost an embodied pragmatic agent who is already physically, affectively, and socially situated in a world defined as a set of practical involvements and affordances (Gibson 1977). The notion of *world* in this context of "being-in-the-world" is clearly relative to the situation of the agent. Another way to say this can be found in pragmatist thinkers like John Dewey, who defines the situation as agent relative – that is, the agent is a constitutive part of what counts as a situation for the agent (Dewey 1938). We refer to this as the 'agentive situation'. As the agent changes, so does the situation, and so does the meaning structure of the world.

This idea is reflected in William James's (1890, II, pp. 291–306) concept of "sub-universes," but is further developed by the phenomenologist Alfred Schutz (1974, pp. 207–259). Schutz explains James's concept of sub-universes in the following way. The experiencing subject does not live in the one unified world of meaning that is defined objectively (in a view from nowhere); rather, the agent lives in multiple realities, sub-universes or finite provinces of meaning. Both James and Schutz suggest that there is a "paramount reality" – the reality of shared everyday life with which we normally engage. This is the world where we work, earn our salary, socialize, enjoy family life, and so forth. But there are also multiple other realities that take us away from everyday reality. If, for example, I read a novel, or go to the theatre or the cinema, or play a video game, I may spend some significant amount of time in a different sort of reality which opens up on the page, on the stage, or on the screen. In such realities, I may not play the role of myself; I may, for example, identify with one or more of the characters presented in these different media. In fantasies, dreams or daydreams, I may more actively play a part as a modified variation of who I take myself to be in everyday paramount reality, rather than the role I usually play.

We can take this idea further by noting that even what Schutz calls paramount reality is not always strongly unified. The role that I play where I work and earn a salary may be quite removed from the role I play in my family life, and that may differ from my pub life among friends. Changing roles can be understood in terms of transitioning from one reality to another. Here we want to appeal to Maria Lugones's (1987, 2003) extremely rich notion of how we may transition from one reality or "world" to another in her concept of "world-traveling."

Lugones allows for the possibility of "weaving" worlds together. Worlds, for her, are cultural constructs, sometimes partial, sometimes incomplete, but necessarily inclusive of other existing agents. Agents can be situated in worlds in ways that escape their understanding.

> In a "world" some of the inhabitants may not understand or hold the particular construction of them that constructs them in that "world." So, there may be "worlds" that construct me in ways that I do not even understand. Or it may be that I understand the construction, but do not hold it of myself. I may not accept it as an account of myself, a construction of myself. And yet, I may be animating such a construction.
>
> (1987, p. 10)

Writing in a context that investigates differences in gender, race and nationality, she takes the plurality of worlds to signal a richness of experience that in some cases we can share with others, and that in some cases can define us as 'outsiders' relative to what might be considered in some places as the paramount reality of White/Anglo organized life. Lugones stresses the tension between an agent's "acquired flexibility in shifting from the mainstream construction of life", where one may be an outsider, "to other constructions of life where she is more or less 'at home'" (1987, p. 3). This flexibility allows for world-traveling, which can be a skill that is willfully exercised ("a skillful, creative, rich, enriching and, given certain circumstances, as a loving way of being and living"), or, in other cases something done out of necessity, unwillingly, forced on the agent by circumstances. In part, the tension concerns the ease (or the difficulty) of transition. In the agentive situation, the degree of ease or difficulty may be due to either the agent, who may be skillful or not, or to the structure of the world, which may be oppressive or supportive, or to the process of integration or coupling that defines the agentive situation.

Traveling includes the possibility of being in two places (worlds) at one time.

> One can "travel" between these "worlds" and one can inhabit more than one of these "worlds" at the very same time. I think that most of us who are outside the mainstream of, for example, the U.S. dominant construction or organization of life are "world travellers" as a matter of necessity and of survival. It seems to me that inhabiting more than one "world" at the same time and "travelling" between "worlds" is part and parcel of our experience and our situation. One can be at the same time in a "world" that constructs one as stereotypically latin, for example, and in a "world" that constructs one as latin. Being stereotypically latin and being simply latin are different simultaneous constructions of persons that are part of different "worlds." One animates one or the other or both at the same time without necessarily confusing them, though simultaneous enactment can be confusing if one is not on one's guard.
>
> (1987, pp. 10–11)

The type of transition that takes place in world-traveling is not just a change in worlds; it entails a change in the agent. More specifically, "worlds" constitute *who* the subject is.

> Those of us who are "world"-travelers have the distinct experience of being different in different "worlds" and of having the capacity to remember other "worlds" and ourselves in them.... The shift from being one person to being a different person is what I call "travel." This shift may not be willful or even conscious, and one may be completely unaware of being different than one is in a different "world," and may not recognize that one is in a different "world."
>
> (1987, p. 11)

Importantly, in Lugones, as in Dewey and Schutz, there is a strong emphasis on the role of the social in constructing the subject. In contrast to Dewey and Schutz, however, she doesn't prioritize the subject's participation in or identification with a particular reality as a resource for information about the agent. Instead, Lugones's plural subject can be understood as a product of the world(s) they inhabit.

Her descriptions of worlds and of traveling are not meant to capture pathology. World traveling is not pathological; it is a way of everyday "normal" life for many people.[1] At the same time, in those contexts where world-traveling is not a skillful, enriching, creative practice, but rather a forced and necessary practice of self-defense, it can easily reflect the dynamics of social pathologies (Lugones 2003, p. 86). Taking this one step further, we propose that the concept can be put to use as a way to understand delusional experience.[2]

Various worlds or multiple realities (and their particular rules or normative structures) are not necessarily commensurable, and my actions or virtual actions are of course different in these different worlds. Usually, however, I can make sense of my behavior in these realities and can understand it from the perspective of everyday reality (or whatever might count as my paramount reality). With respect to playing a video game, I can say, "I didn't really slay a dragon; I was playing a game." There are normally clear transitions as I move from one world to another. In everyday reality I can go to the theatre; once in the theatre, however, I enter a different world. At some level, when I enter into a virtual world, I keep account of the fact that from the perspective of everyday reality, I am playing a game. I can distance myself from the various roles that I might play or fantasize about. In some cases I may become immersed in one of these alternative realities.

> Even in such cases, it is not simply that I adopt an alternative set of beliefs or values. Rather, I may enter into it body and soul, so to speak, or to some varying lesser degree. Indeed, the alternative reality has a certain 'presence' and salience that makes it more than an intellectual exercise. I am in-the-world of the play, the film, the game, etc.; I can get excited and emotional, or remain cool under pressure; I may adopt a certain physical posture, I may act virtually (which itself requires physical movement of my body), and I may engage in such action explicitly or implicitly. (Gallagher 2009, p. 255)

The changes involved in delusions are similarly existential, involving a transformation of background familiarity and of the sense of reality.

Delusions

It seems quite possible that one can travel to or transition into a delusional world just as one can enter into a dream reality, or a fictional reality, or a virtual reality (Gallagher 2009). Like other multiple realities, some delusional realities may be more or less cut off from one's everyday reality. A delusional world may be completely incommensurable with the normal rules that govern one's everyday lifeworld, and it may be such that it offers a different set of affordances. Consider, for example, a description offered by Renee, a schizophrenic patient (Sechehaye 1968; cited in Sass 1992, 118): A jug appeared to her "not as something to hold water and milk, a chair not as something to sit in – but as having lost their names, their functions and meanings; they became 'things' and began to take on life, to exist." As Louis

Sass (1992, p. 109) puts it, the delusional subject "inhabits a world radically alien to that of common sense." Accordingly, when a subject enters into a delusional state, he or she is traveling to and entering into an alternative reality. Unlike other multiple realities, however, this one may be "firmly sustained ... [and] is not one ordinarily accepted by other members of the person's culture or subculture" (DSM-IV). A drama comes to an end when the theatre lights come on. In a firmly sustained delusion, the lights may not come on, although this may vary in degree. One can slip in and out of a delusional reality. One's traveling is not always under one's control.

Worlds created in theatre, film, novels, and games are socially constructed realities; they are made by people and for people, and are understandable to many people. Likewise, in world-traveling, worlds are typically shared worlds. Delusions are more like dreams; they are in some regards idiosyncratic, or as Louis Sass (1994, 2004) puts it, "quasi-solipsistic," although they may share certain culturally bound themes, such as being controlled by others, seeing others as impostors, and so forth. Although delusions are not "for others," they do not exclude others from appearing within the delusional reality.

Delusion involves a radical or structural (or existential) change in the way that the subject relates to everyday reality. Delusional patients sometime report pervasive feelings of strangeness, where everything seems somehow unreal or unfamiliar (Stone & Young 1997, p. 337). In Capgras delusion, for example, although rare, a subject may consider a set of tools as having been replaced by exact doubles (Ellis 1996). The tools remain tools and can be part of the person's everyday reality, but her relation to the tools has been radically reconfigured (see, e.g., Dreyfus 1987; also Kafka 1989). This may be a question of partial transition or what we propose to call *delusional weaving*.[3] In some instances of delusion, it may be more apt to say that the delusional world has been weaved into one's everyday reality, than to say that one has traveled to a completely different world. The difference in the way of putting this, however, reflects how comprehensive or pervasive, or 'firmly sustained' the delusion is or to what extent the subject's interactions with objects in everyday reality are close to normal.

In contrast to the DSM definitions, a delusion is not "a false belief based on incorrect inference about external reality." As we saw, Jaspers points to something much richer – something that the delusional subject experiences and lives through. To consider a delusion to be a false belief, or the result of a dysfunctional introspection about something in everyday (external or objective) reality, is not just overly cognitive; it targets the wrong world. The delusion may not be about external or everyday reality, but may be tied to a different world, in the same way that events that take place in a theatrical play are tied to a fictional reality. My belief that Hamlet killed Polonius, for example, is not a false belief about the objective world.

This can be seen in the accounts that many schizophrenics give of their delusions. Sass (1992, pp. 113, 116) provides some examples.

> In the famous memoir of his psychosis, for example, Daniel Paul Schreber describes what he calls his "so-called delusional system" in terms very different from those used by his psychiatrist. He does not, in fact, make claims about actual characteristics of the objective, external or consensual world – the sort of statements that could be shown to be false by reference to evidence independent of the experiences in question. ... Similarly, another patient described the objects he hallucinated as appearing in "their own private space peculiar to themselves"; the sight of such objects could not, he said, be blocked by real objects, nor could they appear simultaneously with real ones – For a patient to believe such a thing would imply a profoundly altered conception of the everyday physical world – of those laws of gravity, object constancy, or spatial organization that preclude material objects from flying about, materializing instantaneously, or existing inside one's skull. If such were the case, one would expect profound confusion or mistakenness about the physical world; whereas in fact schizophrenics are usually well-oriented and quite capable of practical activity when this is called for.

To consider a delusion as a type of world-traveling, or an entry into an alternative reality, in the sense defined by Schutz, requires that we see it, neither as a set of false beliefs about the objective or everyday world, nor as merely a set of odd beliefs about an alternative world. Rather, it is primarily something experiential; an existential transformation of one's being-in-the-world. Being-in-the-world, as Heidegger defines it, entails a threefold existential structure.

First the is an attunement (*Befindlichkeit*), which Heidegger cashes out as a certain kind of affectivity that manifests itself as mood (Heidegger 1968). The psychiatrist Medard Boss (1979) explains:

> The prevailing attunement is at any given time the condition of our openness for perceiving and dealing with what we encounter. ... What we call moods, feelings, affects, emotions, and states are the concrete modes in which the possibilities for being open are fulfilled. They are at the same time the modes in which this perceptive openness can be narrowed, distorted, or closed off.
>
> (p. 110)

We can think of attunement as a fundamental kind of emotional stance. Naomi Eilan (2000, p. 109), following "Jaspers's sense that the schizophrenic's worlds are different," suggests that at least in some cases, the schizophrenic's occupation of a delusional world comes along with the subject's finding herself affectively attuned in a very idiosyncratic way. Eilan recounts the reports of a schizophrenic who was delusional about bombs falling on her, but not on others around her:

> The bombs were directed at her in a way that made the rest of the world, her family and friends, wholly irrelevant. What brought home the awfulness of this fear, its otherworldliness, was her response to the question of whether her past delusions felt continuous with her current life, with her autobiographical sense of who she is. The answer was that they were completely continuous, and what was clear was that the connection with the present was through the live horror the delusions embodied.
>
> (pp. 111–112)

The continuity or delusional weaving of worlds expressed here between this delusional world and her everyday world suggests that the delusional world was framed not by a mere proposition, or set of beliefs, but by a strong attunement at an affective (emotional) level. The delusional world was more salient than the everyday world inhabited by her relatives and friends. Yet, were her friends to voice their agreement about fearing the bombs, the subject would likely find that odd, as Young (1999) suggests, because they are not part of the delusional world in that way.

The level of weaving multiple worlds, or the detachment from everyday reality (or the feeling of unreality that characterizes many delusions), may vary from one form of delusion and one delusional subject to the next. On the one hand, a Capgras patient who claims that his wife is an impostor when he sees her, in some cases is perfectly accepting of her when he speaks with her on the phone. On the other hand, the delusional feeling is not restricted to misperceiving another as an impostor; it colors experience more generally. Thus, Capgras patients "commonly report more pervasive feelings of strangeness, loss of affective response, and feelings that everything is somehow unreal or unfamiliar" (Stone & Young 1997, p. 337), and "when questioned carefully, they report a more widespread feeling that things have changed in a way that makes them seem not quite right – strange, somehow unfamiliar, almost unreal" (Young 2000, p. 59). A patient who experiences himself as emperor of the world and all-powerful in his delusional world, in his everyday world completely lacks power and is incapable of acting in accordance with his delusional self. The Cotard patient is dead and rotting in the delusional world, but continues to eat and live his life in everyday reality, although they may complain of "feelings of derealisation," and "more general feelings of unreality" (Young & Leafhead 1996, p. 155). In some cases, the delusional world becomes the paramount reality;

and in others, it is more or less detached from everyday reality, which remains paramount to some degree.

Heidegger names a second aspect of being-in-the-world 'understanding' (*Verstehen*), which involves a process in which we are always and already projecting meaning onto things and events, and planning our actions. Certain kinds of attunement, however, can disrupt this kind of projective understanding – paralyzing any action planning, in the case of psychotic depression, for example, or transforming it into a more intense experience, as in the case of anxiety disorder, and in either case making various entities (even of the most ordinary type) more salient than they necessarily are. This kind of aberrant saliency, typically explained by abnormal levels of dopamine (Kapur 2003), may characterize certain features of the delusional world.

The third aspect of being-in-the-world Heidegger associates with 'expression' (*Aussage*). The subject's everyday speech may very well be nonsensical from the perspective of the socially constituted everyday reality that most of us live in most of the time. It may be that the subject expresses the logic of the delusional world from the perspective of that world. From the perspective of our everyday, shared reality, this may very well be (more or less) non-sensible. Still, this is not necessarily reducible to simply having inconsistent or conflicting beliefs – something that, to a certain degree, may occur even in non-pathological subjects. It is more like living in a different world, which may or may not come into conflict with one's everyday world. Alternatively, there may be no coherent logic to it. In the realm of expression, it may be a case of "clang" – the phenomenon in which language drives meaningless associations, based sometimes on rhyming words or similar gestures (Spitzer et al. 2012). Here one might think of a kind of incessant manic traveling, an extreme set of transitions, world to world, in such a way that one never arrives in a coherent world.

Transitional Objects

In the latter case, language may provide both the driver and the vehicle of transition. In less extreme cases, one may ask about how transition between worlds works in the case of delusions. Cermolacce et al. (2018) focus on this question – the contrast between a delusional weaving continuity and a transitional break to a different world. They frame this issue in terms of compossibility (the Bleulerian notion of double bookkeeping) and flexibility, and they look for bridges to facilitate travel between everyday reality and delusional reality. Specifically, they employ the concept of hybrid objects – objects that appear in both everyday (non-delusional) reality and the delusional world. Hybrid objects "can operate as shifters, i.e., as some functional operators letting one switch from one reality to another"

(Cermolacce et al. 2018, p. 1). Hybrid objects have the same meaning in both worlds, as Cermolacce et al. indicate. We suggest that there are non-hybrid transitional objects that facilitate traveling rather than weaving, as we have characterized it[4] – an object that may be found in everyday reality but that leads the subject into the delusion and takes on a special meaning in that delusional world.

There are instances in which different worlds are woven together, such that "persons with delusion may be both here and there at the same time, act and communicate from a distance, feel frequently observed while others are mind-reading their innermost secrets and giving them orders, anticipating their actions, knowing their intentions in advance" (Cermolacce et al. 2018, p. 3). This involves Bleuler's so-called double-bookkeeping, where delusional experience seems to co-exist within the world of non-delusional everyday reality. For Sass (2014) double-bookkeeping means that the delusional subject is doubly oriented to a delusional certitude that stands alongside our shared, practical, everyday world. Patients continue to function in a blended set of realities, and in some sense the delusional aspects remain inconsequential and somewhat flexible, fitting into a functional life with others. Paranoid delusions may be a good example. Cermolacce et al. present a different example, the case of KS, who on the one hand identifies with Christ, is capable of working miracles, and who communicates with Stalin by phone, but on the other hand "lives with his family in a shared reality, having meals, baby-sitting nephews, taking care of sick relatives, being concerned with his father's health and going on holiday with them" (2018, p. 4). His phone operates as a hybrid object since it belongs both to his shared everyday world but also functions as a "hotline" to Stalin. In one instance KS breaks into a nurse's office carrying a rosary and a knife. Cermolacce et al. suggest that these are not hybrid objects since they belong only to the delusional reality and have no place in the shared world with the nurse. They may count as transitional objects, however, leading KS into a more delusional fugue where he is Christ and capable of miracles.

As Cermolacce et al. note, the notion of transitional object was proposed by D. W. Winnicott in a developmental context informed by psychoanalysis. According to Winnicott (1953), a transitional object is an inanimate object, for example a toy or blanket, to which a child attaches as she moves from direct dependence on a caregiver (usually the mother) toward understanding and navigating an independently existing world (Winnicott 1953; Elias et al. 2011). An object can play a transitive role to the extent that it takes on an affective meaning that directs the child toward the world. For Winnicott, in the developmental context, the child imbues objects with affect, in order to both cope with the trauma of disillusionment and dependency and to form attachments with the extra-maternal world. The child regards the object as real, yet it nevertheless holds an element of fantasy.

Taking this idea into the psychiatric context, we can think that the subject may feel moved toward the delusional world, which may in some sense feel inviting and responsive to engagement. One can frame this in terms of Heidegger's notion of attunement, and suggest that, along similar lines to Boss (1979, p. 110), such object-related moods, feelings, affects, emotions are the modes in which one's relation to the everyday world can be redirected, in some cases, closing off the everyday world and opening a more narrow delusional one. For Winnicott, transitional phenomena eventually spread out "over the whole cultural field," informing an intermediate realm between "inner psychic reality and the external world" (1953, p. 91). In a similar way, transitions to a delusional world via transitional objects open up a space where affect and intention are interfused into activities that have meaning in the delusional world, but not in the non-delusional shared everyday world. Cermolacce et al. point to the modulation of affordances that would take place in such a transition. "The interplay of affordances meets the possible polarization of the subject's power over a given object within the relevant reality" (2018, p. 5). While the notion of a hybrid object reflects "a human possibility to be part of several realities at the same time" (Cermolacce et al. 2018, p. 5), the notion of a transitional object reflects the possibility of breaking with everyday reality and traveling to and getting immersed in an alternative world.

Conclusion: Implications for therapy

Cermolacce et al. point to the importance of understanding hybrid objects for the delusional subject in the therapeutic context. Importantly, a hybrid or transitional object can be signified as such, or can actually be a word or phrase, opening up the possibility of symbolically manipulating such an object – manipulating what Heidegger calls expression (*Aussage*) in order to modulate an agent's being-in-the-world.[5] Both hybrid and non-hybrid transitional objects are typically reflected in the patient's narrative, and may offer the possibility of meaningful communication between therapist and patient. In this regard we propose that framing our understanding of delusional experience in terms of multiple realities, Lugones's notion of world-traveling, and our expansion of her concept of weaving can offer not just an alternative explanation to standard accounts of delusion in terms of false or fixed beliefs, but can facilitate a form of therapeutic intervention that starts with the patient's experience as reflected in their narratives. Cermolacce et al. suggest that such interventions may start by supporting the patient's ability to transition from one reality to another. Experimenting with the physical or symbolic manipulation of hybrid or transitional objects may be therapeutically productive. Cermolacce et al. mention KS's phone, which materializes KS's possible power over things, according to the typical affordances of each reality it belongs to" (2018, p. 6; also see Gallagher 2018). More generally they note:

> Clinical examples of the use of the telephone among patients with verbal hallucinations show us how patients lift up their mobile phone to the ear while hearing voices. The evident benefit of such creations ... is to minimize the social impact of verbal hallucination and, while it belongs in the reality of delusion, give it scope to be expressed in the pseudo-normality and shared cultural behavior of appearances, in a (seemingly) shared Reality.
>
> (2018, p. 6)

At the very least, the hybrid object can work as an interface with the delusion in therapeutic contexts, opening up an intersubjective or shared space, allowing interaction between therapist and patient. Such affordance-based therapeutic manipulations may facilitate something approaching a less pathological world-traveling, allowing for a more flexible process where delusions are woven into inconsequential elements of everyday reality, or allowing the patient to cope with traveling between multiple worlds.

Notes

1 This is not to say that everyone who participates in world-traveling does it *well* or "*harmlessly*". World-traveling is something that happens within even some of the smallest human interactions, but Lugones distinguishes between arrogant perception and playful world-traveling to identify more productive instances of travel.

2 Someone may consider this an illegitimate use of the concept, since it is not meant to capture pathology. We're suggesting that the concept of world-traveling can itself travel into a different world. Taking the further step and applying it to delusion can be a form of traveling in the realm of theory formation.

3 Lugones describes weaving as the instance of multiple worlds and aspects of life coming together. It represents the rich, complex plurality of feminist ontology and epistemology; one of the strongest ways Lugones understands the "individual" subject as many. Importantly for Lugones, weaving can still very much involve or be a kind of world-traveling. We build off of her term here to capture a similar instance of "worlds" or delusional realities coming together to create a new world that the subject resides in. However, we distinguish it from the idea of world-traveling in order to highlight the difference between genuine world-traveling and the kind of delusional weaving of worlds that might be experienced by the delusional subject.

4 We want to emphasize here that the distinction between delusional weaving and traveling should strictly be understood in terms of the difference between how the subject is *in-the-world* when multiple worlds come together and when

there is a complete shift in worlds, respectively. Lugones does not distinguish between these two terms in any strong sense.

5 Cermolacce et al. suggest that the language of the delusional patient can be "explored by using discourse analysis tools, collecting narratives about self (Parnas et al., 2005) and world experience (Sass et al., 2017), or focusing on discourse markers (Maj, 2013)" (2018, p. 8; also see Gallagher 2017 for a methodological approach to this type of exploration).

References

American Psychiatric Association (2000). *Diagnostic and Statistical Manual of Mental Disorders, Text Revision.* 4th Edition. (DSM-IV). Washington DC: American Psychiatric Association.

American Psychiatric Association (2013). *Diagnostic and Statistical Manual of Mental Disorders (DSM-5).* 5th Edition. Washington, DC: The American Psychiatric Association.

Boss, M. (1979). *Existential Foundations of Medicine and Psychology* (Trs. S. Conway and A. Cleaves). New York: Jason Aronson.

Campbell, J. (2001). Rationality, meaning, and the analysis of delusion. *Philosophy, Psychiatry, and Psychology*, 8(2–3), 89–100.

Cermolacce, M., Despax, K., Richieri, R., and Naudin, J. (2018). Multiple realities and hybrid objects: A creative approach of schizophrenic delusion. *Frontiers in Psychology*, 9, 107.

Dewey, J. (1938). *Logic: The Theory of Inquiry*. New York: Holt, Rinehart, & Winston.

Dreyfus, H. (1987). Alternative philosophical conceptualizations of psychopathology. In H. A. Durfee, and D. F. T. Rodier (eds.), *Phenomenology and Beyond: The Self and its Language*. Dordrecht: Kluwer Academic, 41–50.

Eilan, N. (2000). On understanding schizophrenia. In D. Zahavi (ed.), *Exploring the Self*. Amsterdam: John Benjamins, 97–113.

Elias, J., Morrow, P. B., Streater, J., Gallagher, S., and Fiore, S. M. 2011. Towards triadic interactions in autism and beyond: Transitional objects, joint attention, and social robotics. *Proceedings of the 55th Annual Meeting of the Human Factors and Ergonomics Society*, vol. 55, no. 1, pp. 1486–1490.

Ellis, H. D. (1996). Delusional misidentification of inanimate objects: A literature review and neuropsychological analysis of cognitive deficits in two cases. *Cognitive Neuropsychiatry*, 1, 27–40.

Gallagher, S. (2009). Delusional realities. In L. Bortolotti, and M. Broome (eds.), *Psychiatry as Cognitive Neuroscience*. Oxford: Oxford University Press, 245–266.

Gallagher, S. (2017). Double phenomenology. *Études Phénoménologiques/Phenomenological Studies*, 1, 29–44.

Gallagher, S. (2018). The therapeutic reconstruction of affordances. *Res Philosophica*, 95(4), 719–736

Gibson, J. J. (1977). The theory of affordances. In R. Shaw, and J. Bransford (eds.), *Perceiving, Acting, and Knowing*. Hillsdale, NJ: Erlbaum, 67–82.

Heidegger, M. (1968). *Being and Time* (Trs. J. Macquarrie, and E. Robinson). New York: Harper and Row.

James, W. (1890). *The Principles of Psychology*. New York: Dover, 1950.

Jaspers, K. (1913/1963). *General Psychopathology* (Trs. J. Hoenig, and M. W. Hamilton). Chicago, IL: University of Chicago Press.

Kafka, J. S. (1989). *Multiple Realities in Clinical Practice.* New Haven: Yale University Press.

Kapur, S. (2003). Psychosis as a state of aberrant salience: A framework linking biology, phenomenology, and pharmacology in schizophrenia. *American Journal of Psychiatry*, 160, 13–23.

Lugones, M. (1987). Playfulness, "world"-travelling, and loving perception. *Hypatia*, 2(2), 3–19.

Lugones, M. (2003). *Pilgrimages/peregrinajes: Theorizing coalition against multiple oppressions.* Maryland: Rowman & Littlefield Publishers.

Maj, M. (2013). Karl Jaspers and the genesis of delusions in schizophrenia. *Schizophrenia Bull.* 39, 242–243. doi: 10.1093/schbul/sbs190

Parnas, J., Møller, P., Kircher, T., Thalbitzer, J., Jansson, L., Handest, P., et al. (2005). EASE: Examination of anomalous self-experience. *Psychopathology*, 38, 236–258. doi: 10.1159/000088441

Sass, L. (1992). Heidegger, schizophrenia and the ontological difference. *Philosophical Psychology*, 5, 109–132.

Sass, L. (1994). *The Paradoxes of Delusion: Wittgenstein, Schreber, and the Schizophrenic Mind.* Ithaca, NY: Cornell University Press.

Sass, L. (2004). Some reflections on the (analytic) philosophical approach to delusion. *Philosophy, Psychiatry, and Psychology*, 11(1), 71–80.

Sass, L. (2014). Delusion and double bookkeeping. In T. Fuchs, T. Breyer, and C. Mundt (eds.), *Karl Jaspers Philosophy and Psychopathology*. Heidelberg: Springer, 125–147.

Sass, L., Pienkos, E., Skodlar, B., Stanghellini, G., Fuchs, T., Parnas, J., et al. (2017). EAWE: Examination of anomalous world experience. *Psychopathology* 50, 10–54. doi: 10.1159/000454928

Schutz, A. (1974). *Collected Papers Vol. 1. The Problem of Social Reality*. Dordrecht: Springer.

Sechehaye, M. (Ed.). (1968). *Autobiography of a Schizophrenic Girl*, (Trans. G. Rubin-Rabson). New York: New American Library.

Spitzer, M., Uehlein, F., Schwartz, M. A., and Mundt, C. (Eds.). (2012). *Phenomenology, Language & Schizophrenia*. Berlin: Springer Science & Business Media.

Stone, T., and Young, A. (1997). Delusions and brain injury: The philosophy and psychology of belief. *Mind and Language*, 12, 327–364.

Winnicott, D. W. (1953). Transitional objects and transitional phenomena: A study of the first not-me possession. *The International Journal of Psychoanalysis*, 34, 89–97.

Young, A. (1999). Delusions. *The Monist*, 82(4), 571–589.

Young, A. (2000). Wondrous strange: The neuropsychology of abnormal beliefs. In M. Coltheart, and M. Davies (eds.), *Pathologies of Belief*. Oxford: Blackwell, 47–73.

Young, A. W., and Leafhead, K. M. (1996). Betwixt life and death: Case studies of the Cotard delusion. In Peter W. Halligan, and John C. Marshall (eds.), *Method in Madness: Case Studies in Cognitive Neuropsychiatry*. London: Routledge, 147–171.

7 Minimal Biological Adaptiveness and the Phenomenology of Delusions in Schizophrenia

Pablo López-Silva

Introduction

Delusions are a complex and severe transdiagnostic phenomena with a higher prevalence in schizophrenia (Rosen et al., 2016, 2020; López-Silva et al., 2022b). From a conceptual point of view, one of the most fundamental debates surrounding the occurrence of delusional phenomena has to do with the discussion about the specific type of mental state instantiated by delusional reports, namely, the typology problem of delusions (López-Silva, 2017; López-Silva & Cavieres, 2022; López-Silva, Núñez de Prado & Fernández, 2022a). The dominant view within this debate – called the *doxastic approach* – conceptualizes delusions as beliefs that are not correct in all particulars or, simply, as *misbeliefs* (Bayne & Pacherie, 2005; McKay & Dennett, 2009; Bortolotti, 2010; López-Silva, 2017; López-Silva, Núñez de Prado, & Fernández, 2022a). Here, the term *belief* refers to a mental state that implements – or embodies – a subject's endorsement of a particular internal or external state of affairs as actual (McKay & Dennett, 2009). Once delusions are characterized as beliefs, a second conceptual issue emerges. This discussion has to do with the question of whether delusional phenomena might carry some kind of benefit for the deluded even if they are accompanied by acute stress or negative feelings (Freud, 1924/1986; McKay & Dennett, 2009; Mishara & Corlett, 2009; López-Silva, 2015; Bortolotti & Lancellotta, 2019; Lancellotta, 2021).

Philosophers and evolutionary psychologists generally agree that beliefs can be *psychologically* and *biologically* adaptive depending on the role they play in a subject's adaptive performance (McKay & Dennett, 2009; Mishara & Corlett, 2009; Coltheart, Langdon & McKay, 2011; Sterzer et al., 2016). Beliefs are *psychologically adaptive* when their adoption helps a subject to deal with – and desirably overcome – psychologically problematic internal or external stimuli (Coltheart, Langdon, & McKay, 2011). Broadly construed, a psychologically problematic stimulus is understood as any stimulus that threatens a subject's self-esteem, self-image, and

DOI: 10.4324/9781003288992-10

self-related representations of the world (see Bentall et al., 2001; Bell, 2003; Lancellotta & Bortolotti, 2021). Beliefs will be *biologically adaptive* when their adoption helps a subject to increase her chances of survival within a specific environment (Millikan, 1993; McKay & Dennett, 2009). Based on this characterization of the relationship between adaptiveness and beliefs, a dominant idea in current literature about delusions is that, while delusional phenomena might be psychologically adaptive, they cannot be biologically adaptive (Roberts, 1992; McKay & Dennett, 2009; Pavlickova et al., 2013; Lancellotta & Bortolotti, 2021; Lancellotta, 2021). True beliefs are a trait that allow humans to adapt successfully to a specific environment for they represent reality in a precise and accurate way. Consequently, false beliefs – such as delusions – would not play any role in increasing adaptational chances.

In this chapter I explore a way in which this discussion might be informed by the phenomenological tradition in psychiatry. By focusing on delusions in schizophrenia, I suggest that this dominant way of understanding the adaptiveness of delusions qua beliefs is not guaranteed. As described by phenomenology, in schizophrenia, the adoption of delusions is accompanied by a number of symptoms – such as auditory-verbal hallucinations (AVH) and other delusions (see Rosen et al., 2016; López-Silva et al., 2022b) – and a number of generalized bodily and quasi-perceptual transformations in the experience of the self, intersubjectivity, and reality (Mayer-Gross et al., 1954; Jaspers, 1963; Mishara, 2010; Sass, 1992; Uhlhaas & Mishara, 2007; Fuchs 2005; Pienkos, Silverstein, & Sass, 2017; López-Silva et al., 2022b). I suggest that, when taking into consideration the phenomenologically rarified conditions in which delusions are adopted in schizophrenia, it is possible to think of delusions as playing a minimal adaptive role from a biological perspective.

The Adaptiveness of Clinical Delusions

During a long time, the discussion about how to understand the adaptive role of psychotic delusions seems to have been hijacked by the psychoanalytic tradition. However, clear attempts to explore this issue are observed within the phenomenological psychopathology tradition (Conrad, 1958; Jaspers 1963) and, more specifically, within the Early Heidelberg School of Psychiatry (Berze & Gruhle, 1929; Mayer-Gross, 1932; see Kendler & Mishara, 2019). The psychoanalytic school pioneered the idea that delusions might play a psychological adaptive role as they were conceptualized as aiming at protecting the *ego* from unbalances in its self-representations through the management of strong negative emotions derived from culturally embedded unconscious conflicts of a sexual nature. Freud suggested that: ‘a delusion is found applied like a patch over the place where originally a rent had appeared in the ego's relation to the external world' (1924/1986, p. 565). In this sense, Freudian psychoanalysis proposes that delusions were one of the ways in which the *ego* protects himself from harming psychological stimuli. Currently, the psychoanalytic tradition has lost part of its explanatory appeal in light of more cognitive and empirically focused approaches to psychopathology (Fuchs, 2022). Nowadays, openly endorsing a doxastic approach, the idea that delusions play a psychological adaptive role has also become a part of the theoretical framework underlying current cognitive neuropsychiatry (Coltheart, Langdon, & McKay, 2011; Bortolotti, 2014). Within this tradition, it is claimed that, in some cases, the adoption of a delusional belief might emerge as a defensive strategy that provides mental relief through the overcoming of external or internal psychological threats to the patient's mental well-being (see Bortolotti, 2014).

Contrasting with the psychological case, it is generally agreed that psychotic delusions cannot be biologically adaptive (Zolotova & Brüne, 2006; McKay & Dennett, 2009; Bortolotti & Lancellotta, 2019; Lancellotta, 2021). The suggestion is not that psychotic delusions are not subjectively desirable. For example, negative emotions such as anger or anxiety might be not subjectively desirable, however, they might play an important role in increasing an individual's chances of survival in her environment. Rather, the suggestion in this context is that biological adaptation requires humans to approximate reality accurately, and only true beliefs can perform this task appropriately. Thus, the beliefs that maximize the survival of the subject in a specific environment are necessarily those that best approximate reality by capturing true states of affairs in the world, that is, true beliefs (Dennett 1971; Fodor 1983; Millikan; 1993). Taking this idea into consideration, beliefs that do not approximate reality in an accurate way cannot increase the subject's chances of survival, and therefore delusional beliefs – as a case of false beliefs – cannot be biologically adaptive (McKay & Dennett, 2009; Bortolotti & Lancellotta, 2019; Lancellotta, 2021). In the following sections, I challenge this idea by proposing that psychotic delusions can play a fundamental biological adaptive role by reestablishing functional levels of interaction between subjects and their environment.

Biological Adaptiveness and Delusions in Schizophrenia

There are a number of problems in the aforementioned formulation of the adaptiveness of delusions; however, in this section I shall only explore one positive argument against it derived from what is actually informed by psychotic patients during the onset of delusion formation in schizophrenia (see Conrad, 1958; Fusar-Poli et al., 2022). Initially, there are two alternatives to counter the dominant formulation. First, we can tie psychological and biological adaptiveness together so that psychological adaptiveness could imply a degree of biological adaptiveness and vice versa; then, if a mental state M is psychologically adaptive, it might be, by extension, also biologically adaptive. Beresford (2012), for example, will claim that the development of psychological defenses would not only affect psychologically adaptive performance, but would also increase survival and reproductive probabilities. In this chapter I explore a second alternative, namely, simply showing directly the fact that some psychotic delusions do play a biological adaptive role without necessarily appealing to their relationship with psychologically adaptive mental states; but first, let me make a preliminary point.

Phenomenal Doxasticism about Delusions

Conscious experiences involve a number of different types of sensory conscious states. We see, hear, smell, taste, and touch things; we also have bodily and affective states of different kinds. All these states enjoy a distinctive *phenomenal character*, that is, *there is something that it is like* to be in those states or, in other words, they *feel* in a distinctive way (Nagel, 1974). Consciousness also includes cognitive experiences such as thoughts and beliefs. As explained by Bayne and Montague (2011), a number of authors within the analytic philosophy tradition accept the idea that the domain of phenomenology can be extended beyond the sensory and claim that conscious thoughts and beliefs also possess some kind of phenomenality. In other words, the idea is that there is *something that is like* to think that P, or believe that T. As Strawson (1994) claims:

> [T]he experience of seeing red and the experience of now seeming to understand this very sentence, and of thinking that nobody could have had different parents ... all fall into the vast category of experiential episodes that have a certain qualitative character for those who have them as they have them.
>
> (p. 194)

Most doxastic argumentation – the idea that delusions are beliefs – focuses on third person attribution of delusions to a subject, inheriting a lot of ideas from interpretivism and functionalism about the mind (see Bortolotti, 2010; López-Silva, Núñez de Prado & Fernández, 2022a). From this point of view, it is not easy to see how delusions might be referred to as types of belief without appealing to disembodied and impersonal evaluative epistemic conditions such as justification, rationality, action-guidance, and the like (López-Silva, 2017). The problem with this narrow content-focused approach to the doxastic question is its tendency to isolate delusional phenomena from the experiential context in which they are adopted, overlooking the generalized mutation of the subject's field of consciousness in which these phenomena are adopted (Mishara & Zaytseva, 2019; Fayaerts et al., 2021). Importantly, these seem to be the mark of psychotic delusions, and therefore, we cannot understand delusional phenomena without them. Therefore, rather than purely focusing on the '*what*' of delusional beliefs (content), it is necessary to incorporate the '*how*' of delusions into the discussion, namely, the way in which psychopathological phenomena are experienced by subjects in a first-personal sense (Jaspers, 1963; Sass & Byrom, 2015). Here the incorporation of the phenomenological tradition is fundamental due to its focus on delusions as a phenomenon on its subjective and lived dimension, namely, on *what it is like* to have a delusion (Sass & Byrom, 2015).

In the remainder of this chapter, I shall endorse the idea that there is *something that is like to have a certain belief* that is different from what it is like to have a belief with a different content – in other words, the idea that beliefs are dispositional states accompanied by phenomenal features. I call this view *Phenomenal Doxasticism* (see Kriegel, 2015; Clutton, 2018). Endorsing Kriegel's (2015) cognitive phenomenological approach to beliefs, Clutton (2018, p.4) suggests that: 'beliefs are dispositions to have certain intentional, occurrent mental states whose phenomenal character is that of "judging that P." Specifically, on this view, S believes that P iff S is disposed to immediately judge that P when P-entertaining triggers obtain' (Clutton, 2018, p. 4). When we judge that P (consider P to be true), we feel a sense of mental affirming expressed in phenomenological conviction, and those epistemic feelings constitute – among many others – the phenomenal mark of cognitive states such as thoughts and beliefs. From this point of view, Phenomenal Doxasticism about delusions will be the view that delusions are a type of phenomenally conscious mental states, and, in consequence, phenomenological descriptions about them are not only in place, but they are necessary in order to understand the phenomenon appropriately. By endorsing Phenomenal Doxasticism about delusions, we can find a way in which the phenomenological tradition might interact with the way in which other traditions have thought about delusions over the years. In addition, we now are able to incorporate the *how* of delusions into the discussion about whether they can be biologically adaptive.

Pre-delusional Alterations in Schizophrenia

Delusions in schizophrenia do not arise *out of the blue*. Rather, their adoption is preceded by a period characterized by a number of affective and perceptual changes in the way patients experience themselves and the world (Conrad, 1958; Jaspers, 1963; Fuchs, 2005; López-Silva, 2018). This period may last days, weeks, months or even years (Conrad, 1958; Payne, 2013). During this period:

> Patients feel uncanny and that there is something suspicious afoot. Everything gets a new meaning. The environment is somehow different –not to a gross degree –, perception is unaltered in itself but there is some change which envelops everything with a subtle, pervasive and strangely uncertain light. ... Something seems in the air which the patient cannot account for, a distrustful, uncomfortable, uncanny tension invades him.
>
> (Jaspers, 1963, p. 98)

This period can be understood as an *incubation phase*, where psychotic symptoms are not yet present in the patient's consciousness, but they seem to be in subtle development. In this sense, the adoption of a delusional belief shows the final stage of a long period of perceptual and affective alterations in the way the external world and subjectivity is experienced (López-Silva, 2015; Fusar-Poli et al., 2022). On the perceptual side, this prodromal period is characterized by a general transformation in the field of awareness of the world without affecting the objects of perception but the way they are presented to subjects (Jaspers, 1963). A patient claims that 'everything is strange ... , everything is somehow different' (Sass, 1992, p. 46). In this way, the whole surrounding environment becomes alien, puzzling, and mysterious. A subject reports that during this period 'wherever you are looking, everything looks unreal' and that 'people went down the street like in a puppet theatre' (Gross & Huber, 1972). Another patient claims that 'when you go somewhere, everything seems already set up for you like in a theatre – it's really eerie, and you get terribly frightened' (Fuchs, 2005, p. 134). During recent years, all these phenomenological changes in perception have been associated with significant alterations in brain functions (Fusar-Poli, Allen & McGuire, 2008), structure (Fusar-Poli et al., 2012), and neurochemistry (Fusar-Poli et al., 2011).

Now, on the affective side, the period preceding the adoption of delusions in psychosis is characterized by high rates of affective instability (Strauss et al., 2013) and mood instability (Broome et al., 2012). During this period, patients also report high rates of anxiety and depressive states (Broome et al., 2005, 2012; Fusar-Poli et al., 2022). These rates tend to enhance reactivity to negative stimuli, increasing negative affectivity and prompting a generalized sense of emotional dyscontrol (Aiello et al., 2012; Buckley et al., 2009; Strauss et al., 2013). All these pre-psychotic affective alterations color the way in which patients experience the world and themselves with an overwhelming negative and confusing character (Gibbs; 2000; Fuchs, 2013). It is important to note that all these disturbed dimensions of affectivity seem to have a crucial doxastic role in the psychogenesis of some delusions, given the general role they have in the process of belief and thought formation (O'Driscoll, Laing & Mason, 2014). All these dimensions manifest themselves subjectively in the patient's life as an intense, overwhelming, confusing, and stressful affective experience of the world and themselves, leading – in conjunction with other deficits – to the adoption of delusional beliefs (Fusar-Poli et al., 2022). About this, Marwaha et al. (2013, p. 6) claim that 'the sense that emotional experiences are out of one's personal control may prompt a search for meaning that may find explanations in terms of external influence', a suggestion that is consistent with the subjective structure of a number of delusions such as thought insertion, alien control, thought withdrawal, among many others.

Psychotic Delusions as Biological Adaptive Devices: A Brief Proposal

In order to understand *how* psychotic delusions can play a biological adaptive role, we need to take into consideration the role they play within the affectively and perceptually rarified context in which they are adopted. In staying alert to adaptively relevant elements of their surrounding environment – such as potentially dangerous stimuli, sources of nourishment, and reproductive opportunities – humans try to maintain a minimal degree of stable and predictable psychological and behavioral interchange with it. This minimal level of socially functional engagement with the environment will allow physical and psychological adaptation through the participation of ecological niches (Walsh, 2015), creating a socially shared world implicitly experienced as a background for every conscious experience (Blankenburg, 1980). Disturbances in this minimal degree of interaction might affect a subject's adaptive performance and, therefore, the subject's chances of survival.

Problematically, all the aforementioned alterations in affectivity and perception disrupt the quality of this interaction with the environment, decreasing the subject's chances of survival. In contrast with their manifestation in non-pathological cases, phenomenal consciousness, self-consciousness, and inter-subjective consciousness in psychosis manifest themselves as very confusing and deeply fragmented states (Uhlhaas & Silverstein, 2005). The unity and coherence of the affective and perceptual experience of the patient's inner and outer world breaks down, and finally, the experience of the whole world becomes gradually incoherent, disconnected, and disharmonious (Doniger et al., 2001; Keefe & Kraus, 2009). Gradually, patients start having a highly unpredictable experience of their social, inner, and physical worlds (Kapur, 2003). The generalized feelings of uncertainty and lack of control that pervade the different dimensions of patients' consciousness during the period preceding the adoption of delusions gradually lead them to lose their behavioral connection with the environment. Ratcliffe (2013) reports that during this period, physical and mental objects do not invite any type of activity, so patients stop experiencing themselves as the agents of their own mental and physical lives. Thus, a feeling of practical disengagement and passivity progressively pervades their experience of the world and themselves (Fusar-Poli et al., 2022).

However, this period is characterized by not only a gradual loss of behavioral connection with the environment, but also by a progressive loss of psychological connection with the intersubjective world (Van Duppen, 2017). As we all know, we humans do not only inhabit a shared physical but also a world replete with socially shared meanings where the functional manipulation of these meanings seems to be a fundamental adaptive advantage (Blankenburg, 1980; Scarantino, 2003; Stanghellini, 2004). Arguably, normal perceptual abilities might not be as useful as they are if they did not incorporate these shared meanings into their deployment. Perceiving a bunch of wooden parts attached to each other is adaptively different from perceiving a *chair as a chair*. Now, in the midst of the confusing and unpredictable experience of inner and outer reality that precedes the adoption of delusions, physical and mental objects seem to gain random and peculiar meanings. Fuchs (2005) reports the case of a patient who claims that during this period: 'the sight of a limping man on the street may suddenly evoke the impression of the devil hunting the patient. … [T]he stroke of a bell may announce his imminent death' (p. 134). In this period, patients lose the familiar meanings of the perceived objects and situations, and this leads to a fundamental disruption of the phenomenological constitution of the patient's intersubjective world. Patients feel like they are in a foreign country unable to grasp the shared language and social meanings of their new community (Klosterkötter & Gross, 1988). The upshot of all these changes is that patients gradually lose the feeling of inhabiting a shared intersubjective world (Ratcliffe, 2013).

Taking the general set of transformations experienced by patients during the period preceding the adoption of delusional beliefs, I propose that some delusions in the context of schizophrenia would be adopted as a way of re-establishing a minimal degree of phenomenological, cognitive, and behavioral order that allows the patients to approximate their reality in a better way – in comparison with the way they do during the pre-delusional period. In this sense, the reestablishment of this minimal degree of interaction would secure the necessary condition for a person to develop a functional adaptive behaviour. Contrasting with the way in which a subject's mental states are deployed during the period preceding the adoption of delusions, patients reporting actual delusions can distinguish between different agents (a spouse being replaced by an alien, a certain entity inserting thoughts into their mind, the 'organization' trying to kill them, etc.) and establish basic predictable causal connections between different aspects of their delusions. For example, patients suffering from thought insertion establish a causal link between the inserted thought and its external author with a high degree of certainty (López-Silva, 2018). In this sense, the crystallization of a delusion might help to recover *some* sense of agency over the part of reality that is no longer psychotized. The fixation of the delusion in a subject's mind allows her to move from a generally rarefied reality to a state where only some pieces of her mind are altered (Conrad, 1958; Jaspers, 1963). This allows a subject to bring back true beliefs that help her to act more successfully in the environment. I shall call this the *minimal biological adaptiveness of delusions*.

From this point of view, some psychotic delusions represent an attempt to re-establish some of the many aspects of the psychotic mind that break down in the stages that precede the adoption of the delusion in schizophrenia and, through the reappearance of clear true beliefs in the subject's mind, the adoption of delusions would allow subjects to act purposely in their environment. Here, the adoption of a delusional belief would increase the subject's chances of survival within his environment, for this mental act would help him to reestablish a minimally organized degree of interaction with the environment. About this, Mishara & Corlett (2009) suggest that: 'Delusions are not primarily a defensive reaction to protect the self, but involve a "reorganization" of the patient's experience to maintain behavioural interaction with the environment despite the underlying disruption to perceptual binding processes' (p. 531). The pervasive feeling of uncertainty experienced by patients – along with other factors, such as cognitive and affective impairments – drives the adoption of delusional beliefs as an attempt to render the world more psychologically and behaviourally predictable, and therefore, approachable. The adoption of delusional beliefs might allow the reorganization of part of the experience of the world into a more or less unitary *gestalt* that was disrupted during the period preceding this action. The idea is that in the midst of this phenomenologically disorganized experience of the world, patients search for some 'fixed point' to which they can cling, and the delusional belief is the outcome of that search (Mishara & Corlett, 2009). Finally, it is important to note that McKay and Dennett's proposal seems to rely on a problematic idea, namely, that epistemic accuracy is a necessary condition for a certain belief to be biologically adaptive. I disagree with this, for as Haselton and Nettle (2006, p. 63) rightly point out, '[t]he human mind shows good design, although it is design for fitness maximization, not truth preservation'. Adaptation is not about truth, but survival, and sometimes – as what patients' reports seem to show – the human cognitive system might sacrifice doxastic accuracy in favour of biological adaptation. When considering the role that the adoption of delusions in schizophrenia play in re-unifying a subject's phenomenal field of awareness, it is plausible to think about these delusions as having a minimal biologically adaptive role.

Concluding Remarks

Delusions are the mark of psychosis par excellence, their occurrence leading to a number of empirical and conceptual debates. This chapter has engaged with the discussion about how to understand the adaptive role that delusions might play in a subject's mind in the context of schizophrenia. Contrasting with the dominant view primarily defended by McKay and Dennett, here I have suggested that, when considering the different phenomenological alterations that characterize the period preceding the adoption of some delusional beliefs, this psychopathological phenomenon might be regarded as minimally biologically adaptive in virtue of the way it allows the reorganization of the patient's experiential world and the way it allows the reincorporation of the true beliefs into the subject's field of awareness. The guiding idea is that delusions in schizophrenia might help to restore a minimal degree of interaction between a subject and his environment through the stabilization of the subject's phenomenal field of awareness, and therefore, the adoption of certain delusions might increase the chances of survival of a subject within a chaotic and experientially rarified environment. At his point, it is important to note that further research is needed in order to clarify the way in which delusions might act as biologically adaptive devices. For example, this type of adaptiveness might work for only short periods of time. In addition, it is important to note that here I have limited my proposal to those delusions that are adopted in the midst of a generally rarified experience of the world and the self in schizophrenia. Therefore, the application of my proposal to other types of delusions remains an open question.

Acknowledgements

This work was supported by the project FONDECYT regular n° 1221058 'The architecture of delusions' granted by the Chilean National Agency for Research and Development (ANID) of the Government of Chile, and the Project FACSO 2/2021 granted by the Universidad de Valparaíso, Chile. I would like to thank to Tim Bayne, Joel Smith, Cherise Rosen, Aaron Mishara, Geraldine Ellwanger, and my students from the Psychology Research Seminar 2022 for insightful comments on the early stages of this work.

References

Aiello, G., Horowitz, M., Hepgul, N., Pariante, C. M., & Mondelli, V. (2012). Stress abnormalities in individuals at risk for psychosis: A review of studies in subjects with familial risk or with “at risk” mental state. *Psychoneuroendocrinology*, 37, 1600–1613.

American Psychiatric Association. (2013). *Diagnostic and Statistical Manual of Mental Disorders (DSM-5®)*. Washington, DC: American Psychiatric Pub.

Bayne, T. & Montague, M. (2011). *Cognitive Phenomenology*. Oxford: Oxford University Press.

Bayne, T. & Pacherie, E. (2005). In defence of the doxastic conception of delusion. *Mind & Language*, 20(2), 163–188.

Bell, D. (2003). *Paranoia*. Cambridge, UK: Icon.

Beresford, T. (2012). *Psychological Adaptive Mechanisms: Ego Defense Recognition and Research*. Oxford: OUP.

Berze, J., & Gruhle, H. W. (1929). *Psychologie der Schizophrenie*. Berlin: Julius Springer.

Bentall, R. P., Corcoran, R., Howard, R., Blackwood, N., & Kinderman, P. (2001). Persecutory delusions: A review and theoretical integration. *Clinical Psychology Review*, 21, 1143–1192.

Blankenburg, W. (1980). Anthropological and ontoanalytical aspects of delusion. *Journal of Phenomenological Psychology*, 11(1), 97.

Bortolotti, L. (2014). The epistemic innocence of motivated delusions. *Consciousness and Cognition*, 33, 490–499.

Bortolotti, L. (2010). *Delusions and other Irrational Beliefs*. Oxford: Oxford University Press.

Broome, M. R., Day, F., Valli, I. et al. (2012). Delusional ideation, manic symptomatology and working memory in a cohort at clinical high-risk for psychosis: A longitudinal study. *European Psychiatry*, 27, 258–263.

Broome, M. R., Woolley, J. B., Tabraham, P. et al. (2005). What causes the onset of psychosis? *Schizophrenia Research*, 79, 23–34.

Buckley, P. F., Miller, B. J., Lehrer, D. S., & Castle, D. J. (2009). Psychiatric comorbidities and schizophrenia. *Schizophrenia Bulletin*, 35, 383–402.

Clutton, P. (2018). A new defence of doxasticism about delusions: The cognitive phenomeno- logical defence. *Mind & Language*, 33(2), 198–217. https://doi.org/10.1111/mila.12164

Coltheart, M., Langdon, R., & McKay, R. (2011). Delusional belief. *Annual Review of Psychology*, 62, 271–298.

Conrad, K. (1958). *Die beginnende Schizophrenie*. Stuttgart, Germany: Thieme Verlag.

Dennett, D. C. (1971) Intentional systems. *Journal of Philosophy*, 68(2), 87–106.

Doniger, G. M., Silipo, G., Rabinowicz, E. F., Snodgrass, J. G., & Javitt, D. C. (2001). Impaired sensory processing as a basis for object-recognition deficits in schizophrenia. *The American Journal of Psychiatry*, 158(11), 1818–1826.

Feyaerts, J., Kusters, W., Van Duppen, Z., Vanheule, S., Myin-Germeys, I., & Sass, L. (2021). Uncovering the realities of delusional experience in schizophrenia: A qualitative phenomenological study in Belgium. *Lancet Psychiatry* 8(9), 784–796.

Fodor, J. A. (1983). *The Modularity of Mind*. Cambridge, MA: MIT Press.
Freud, S. (1924/1986). Neurosis and Psychosis (J. Strachey, Trans.) In A. Freud (Ed.), *The Essentials of Psychoanalysis: The Definitive Collection of Sigmund Freud's Writing*. London: Penguin.
Fuchs, T. (2022). Understanding as explaining: How motives can become causes. *Phenomenology and the Cognitive Sciences*. https://doi.org/10.1007/s11097-022-09839-1
Fuchs, T. (2013). The Phenomenology of Affectivity. In K. Fulford, M. Davies, R. Gipps, G. Graham, J. Sadler, G. Stanghellini & T. Thornton (Eds.), *The Oxford Handbook of Philosophy and Psychiatry* (221–239). Oxford: OUP.
Fuchs, T. (2005). Delusional mood and delusional perception. A phenomenological analysis. *Psychopathology*, 38, 133–139. https://doi.org/10.1159/000085843.
Fusar-Poli, P., Estradé, A., Stanghellini, G., Venables, J., Onwumere, J., Messas, G., Gilardi, L., Nelson, B., Patel, V., Bonoldi, I., Aragona, M., Cabrera, A., Rico, J., Hoque, A., Otaiku, J., Hunter, N., Tamelini, M. G., Maschião, L. F., Puchivailo, M. C., Piedade, V. L., Kéri, P., Kpodo, L., Sunkel, C., Bao, J., Shiers, D., Kuipers, E., Arango, C., & Maj, M. (2022). The lived experience of psychosis: A bottom-up review co-written by experts by experience and academics. *World Psychiatry*, 21(2), 168–188. https://doi.org/10.1002/wps.20959. PMID: 35524616; PMCID: PMC9077608. CopyDownload.nbib
Fusar-Poli, P., Radua, J., McGuire, P., & Borgwardt, S. (2012). Neuroanatomical maps of psychosis onset: Voxel-wise metaanalysis of antipsychotic-naive VBM studies. *Schizophrenia Bulletin*, 38, 1297–1307.
Fusar-Poli, P., Howes, O. D., Allen, P., et al. (2011). Abnormal prefrontal activation directly related to pre-synaptic striatal dopamine dysfunction in people at clinical high risk for psychosis. *Molecular Psychiatry*, 16, 67–75.
Fusar-Poli, P., Allen, P., & McGuire, P. (2008). Neuroimaging studies of the early stages of psychosis: A critical review. *European Psychiatry*, 23, 237–244.
Gibbs, P. (2000). Thought insertion and the inseparability thesis. *Philosophy, Psychiatry, and Psychology*, 7(3), 195–202.
Gross, G. & Huber, G. (1972). Sensorische Störungen bei Schizophrenien. *Archiv für Psychiatrie und Nervenkrankheiten*, 216, 119–130.
Haselton, M. G. & Nettle, D. (2006). The paranoid optimist: An integrative evolutionary model of cognitive biases. *Personality and Social Psychology Review*, 10(1), 47–66.
Jaspers, K. (1963). *General Psychopathology* (7th edition). Manchester: Manchester University Press.
Kapur, S. (2003). Psychosis as a state of aberrant salience: A framework linking biology, phenomenology, and pharmacology in schizophrenia. *American Journal of Psychiatry* 160(1), 13–23.
Keefe, R. S. E. & Kraus, M. S. (2009). Measuring memory-prediction errors and their consequences in youth at risk for schizophrenia. Annals of the Academy of Medicine, Singapore, 38(5), 414–416. *Bulletin*, 40(2), 278–286.
Kendler, K. S. & Mishara, A. (2019). The prehistory of schneider's first-rank symptoms: Texts from 1810 to 1932. *Schizophrenia Bulletin*, 45(5), 971–990. https://doi.org/10.1093/schbul/sbz047

Klosterkötter, J. & Gross, G. (1988). Wahrnehmungsfundierte Wahnwahrnehmungen. In F. Böcker &W. Weig (Eds.), *Aktuelle Kernfragen in der Psychiatrie*. Berlin, Heidelberg: Springer. https://doi.org/10.1007/978-3-642-73082-5_11

Kriegel, U. (2015). *The Varieties of Consciousness*. Oxford: Oxford University Press.

Lancellotta, E. (2021). Is the biological adaptiveness of delusions doomed? *Review of Philosophy and Psychology*. https://doi.org/10.1007/s13164-021-00545-6

Lancellotta, E. & Bortolotti, L. (2021). Are clinical delusions adaptive?. *Wiley Interdisciplinary Reviews: Cognitive Science*, 10, e1502. https://doi.org/10.1002/wcs.1502

López-Silva, P. & Cavieres, A. (2022). El delirio psicótico como objeto de estudio multidisciplinar para la filosofía de la mente. *Sophia*, 33, 71–90.

López-Silva, P., Núñez de Prado, M., & Fernández, V. (2022a). Sobre Doxasticismos y Anti-Doxasticismos: Hacia un Mapeo del Problema Tipológico de los Delirios. *Resistances: Journal of Philosophy of History*, 3(6), 1–16. https://doi.org/10.46652/resistances.v3i6.95

López-Silva, P. Harrow, M., Jobe, T., Tufano, M., Hallow, H., & Rosen, C. (2022b). A 20-year prospective study of thought insertion, thought withdrawal and thought broadcasting and their relationship to auditory verbal hallucinations. *Schizophrenia Research*. https://doi.org/10.1016/j.schres.2022.07.005

López-Silva, P. (2018). Mapping the psychotic mind: A review on thought insertion. *Psychiatric Quarterly*, 89(1), 957–968. https://doi.org/10.1007/s11126-018-9593-4

López-Silva, P. (2017). The typology problem and the doxastic approach to delusions. *Filosofía Unísinos*, 17(2), 202–211.

López-Silva, P. (2015). Schizophrenia and the place of egodystonic states in the aetiology of thought insertion. *The Review of Philosophy & Psychology*, 7(3), 577–594.

Mayer-Gross, W., Slater, E., & Roth, M. (1954). *Clinical Psychiatry* (1st, 2nd and 3rd editions). London: Baillière, Tindall & Cassell.

Mayer-Gross, W. (1932). In Geisteskrankheiten, H. D. (Ed.), *Die Klinik der Schizophrenie*. Berlin.

Marwaha, S. Broome, M., Bebbington, P., Kuipers, E., & Freeman, D. (2013). Mood instability and psychosis: Analyses of British National Survey Data. *Schizophrenia Bulletin*, 40(2), 269–277. https://doi.org/10.1093/schbul/sbt149

Mishara, A. L. & Zaytseva, Y. (2019). Hallucinations and Phenomenal Consciousness. In Stanghellini, G., Raballo, A., Broome, M. R., Fernandez, A. V., Fusar-Poli, P., Rosfort, R. (Eds.), *Oxford Handbook of Phenomenological Psychopathology*. Oxford: Oxford University Press.

Mishara, A. L. (2010). Klaus Conrad (1905–1961): Delusional mood, psychosis, and beginning schizophrenia. *Schizophrenia Bulletin* 36(1), 9–13.

Mishara, A. L., & Corlett, P. (2009). Are delusions biologically adaptive? Salvaging the doxastic shear pin. *Behavioral and Brain Sciences*, 32, 530–531.

McKay, R., & Dennett, D. (2009). The evolution of misbelief. *Behavioural and Brain Sciences*, 32(6), 493–561.

Millikan, R. G. (1993) *White Queen Psychology and other Essays for Alice*. Cambridge: MIT Press.

Nagel, T. (1974). What is it like to be a bat?, *Philosophical Review*, LXXXIII, 435–450.

O'Driscoll, C. Laing, J., & Mason, O. (2014). Cognitive emotion regulation strategies, alexithymia and dissociation in schizophrenia, a review and meta-analysis. *Clinical Psychology Review*. https://doi.org/10.1016/j.cpr.2014.07.002

Payne, R. (2013). *Speaking to my Madness*. USA: CreateSpace.

Pavlickova, H., Varese, F., Smith, A., Myin-Germeys, I., Turnbull, O. H., & Bentall, R. P. (2013). The dynamics of mood and coping in bipolar disorder: longitudinal investigations of the inter-relationship between affect, self-esteem and response styles. *PLoS One*, 8(4), e62514.

Pienkos, E., Silverstein, S., & Sass, L. (2017). The phenomenology of anomalous world experience in schizophrenia: A qualitative study. *Journal of Phenomenological Psychology*, 48(2), 188–213.

Ratcliffe, M. (2013). Delusional Atmosphere and the Sense of Unreality. In Stanghellini, G. & Fuchs, T. (Eds.), *One Century of Karl Jaspers' General Psychopathology* (229–244). Oxford: Oxford University Press.

Roberts, G. (1992). The origin of delusions. *The British Journal of Psychiatry*, 16f1, 298–308.

Rosen, C. et al. (2020). The role of inner speech on the association between childhood adversity and 'hearing voices'. *Psychiatry Research*, 286 (April), 112866. https://doi.org/10.1016/j.psychres.2020.112866.

Rosen, C., Jones, N., Chase, K. A., Gin, H., Grossman, L. S., & Sharma, R. P. (2016). The intrasubjectivity of self, voices and delusions: A phenomenological analysis. *Psychosis*, 8(4), 357–368. https://doi.org/10.1080/17522439.2016.1162839.

Sass, L. & Byrom, G. (2015). Phenomenological and neurocognitive perspectives on delusions: A critical overview. *World Psychiatry*, 14, 164–173.

Sass, L. A. (1992). *Madness and Modernism: Insanity in the Light of Modern Art, Literature, and Thought*. New York: Basic Books.

Scarantino, A. (2003). Affordances explained. *Philosophy of Science*, 70(5), 949–961.

Stanghellini, G. (2004). *Disembodied Spirits and De-animated Bodies*. The Psychopathology of Common Sense. Oxford: Oxford University Press.

Sterzer, P., Mishara, A. L., Voss, M., & Heinz, A. (2016). Thought insertion as a self-disturbance: An integration of predictive coding and phenomenological approaches. *Frontiers in Human Neuroscience*, 10, 502.

Strauss, G. P., Kappenman, E. S., Culbreth, A. J., Catalano, L. T., Lee, B. G., & Gold. J. M. (2013). Emotion regulation abnormalities in schizophrenia: Cognitive change strategies fail to decrease the neural response to unpleasant stimuli. *Schizophrenia Bulletin*, 39, 872–883

Strawson, G. (1994). *Mental Reality*. Cambridge, MA: MIT Press.

Uhlhaas, P. J., & Mishara, A. L. (2007). Perceptual anomalies in schizophrenia: Integrating phenomenology and cognitive neuroscience. *Schizophrenia Bulletin*, 33(1), 142–156.

Uhlhaas, P. J., & Silverstein, S. M. (2005). Perceptual organization in schizophrenia spectrum disorders: Empirical research and theoretical implications. *Psychological Bulletin*, 131(4), 618–632.

Walsh, D. M. (2015). *Organisms, Agency, and Evolution*. Cambridge: Cambridge University Press.
Van Duppen, Z. (2017). The intersubjective dimension of schizophrenia. *Philosophy, Psychiatry, and Psychology*, 24(4), 399–418.
Zolotova, J., & Brüne, M. (2006) Persecutory delusions: Reminiscence of ancestral hostile threats? *Evolution and Human Behavior*, 27(3), 185–927.

8 An Active Inference Account of the Cotard Delusion of Inexistence

Philip Gerrans

Introduction

This chapter uses the Cotard delusion as a case study of an approach to the mind inspired by an "active inference" approach to cognition. The concept of active inference, detached from biophysical and mathematical formulations, effectively makes cognition a form of regulatory action (Pezzulo, Rigoli et al. 2015; Barrett, Quigley et al. 2016; Kirchhoff, Parr et al. 2018; Corcoran, Pezzulo et al. 2020; Parr, Pezzulo et al. 2022). On this view, hormonal and electrochemical signalling, homeostatic reflex arcs, perception, sensorimotor processing and higher-level cognition are part of a continuous process of systemic regulation (Huebner and Schulkin 2022). Extending the application of this idea from basic homoestatic regulation to regulation using higher levels of cognition and planning produces the notion of *allostatic* active inference. A feature of the allostatic active inference conception is that *all* activity is ultimately measured against a model of the self that predicts how interoceptive (basic internal bodily) and affective feeling states are affected by action (Barrett, Quigley et al. 2016; Corcoran and Hohwy 2017). As Anil Seth put it:

> *mental representations of selfhood* [the self-model]*are ultimately grounded in representations of the body, with the internal physiological milieu providing a primary reference* – a '**material me**' [13] – that supports adaptive interaction with the environment.
>
> (my italics; Seth 2013)

This idea has consequences for many psychiatric disorders characterised by altered self-awareness. In this chapter I discuss the relationship between two disorders, depersonalisation and the Cotard delusion. I compare the active *inference* account to neuropsychiatric two factor accounts that treat the Cotard delusion as an hypothesis adopted to explain the experience of depersonalisation. I disagree, but the concepts of self-modelling and active

DOI: 10.4324/9781003288992-11

inference are required to explain the nature of that disagreement as well as the areas of overlap between the two accounts.

Depersonalisation is a disorder in which the self model is intact but affective experiences are not annexed to it, leading the subject to feel "as if" she does not exist. It is not the lack of affective response per se that produces depersonalisation but the fact that the self model *predicts* affective consequences of regulatory action. It is important to this account that other predictions generated by different levels and dimensions of self-modelling (interoceptive and narrative) are *intact* in depersonalisation. So the depersonalised subject whose "sensorium is otherwise intact" feels estranged or detached from experience. I shall argue that in the Cotard delusion the self model corrodes or disintegrates. The result is the subject no longer experiences herself as a source and target of active inference. Her sensations are not integrated and unified by the self model, and she cannot predict the consequences of regulatory action. So she is correct to say that what she understood as source and target of predictable regulation no longer exists.

This account differs from influential two factor explanations of the relationship between the depersonalisation experience and the Cotard delusion perfectly encapsulated by Alexandre Billon. He says:

> [there is] almost perfect one to one correspondence between the typical self-oriented delusions of Cotard patients and the complaints of depersonalised patients: the latter just seem to be Cotard patient's delusions prefaced by a neutralising 'it is as if.' The Cotard syndrome can thus be characterised as the delusional form of depersonalisation, depersonalisation being, conversely, the 'as if' form of the Cotard syndrome.
>
> (Billon 2016)

On this view, depersonalisation experience is the essence of Cotard delusion (the first factor), and the second factor in delusion formation consists in a metacognitive abnormality that means the subject *endorses* her experience. Instead of saying 'it is "as if" I do not exist' she forms the belief that she does not exist.

This is an extremely elegant explanation, and as we shall see, it has neuropsychiatric credentials with recent neuropsychiatric explanations proposing that the first factor (depersonalization experience) is hypoactivity or abnormal functioning of the insular cortex.

Below I outline an account of insula function grounded in allostatic active inference theory that provides an alternative account of the relationship between depersonalisation and the Cotard delusion. The short answer is that the insula cortex is a *hub* of hierarchical self-modelling. Depersonalisation and Cotard delusion are different but related forms of dysfunction of this insula-based self-modelling process. In depersonalisation, the typical cause is *dissociative deaffectualisation* that selectively deactivates the *anterior* insula but leaves the rest of the substrates of the self-modelling hierarchy intact. In Cotard delusion, the primary cause is *catastrophic dyshomeostasis*, which affects insula function by a different route and destroys self-modelling with pervasive, cascading consequences for regulatory functions. This is why Cotard delusion is typically part of a syndrome of intractable anomalous bodily experiences (Gerrans 2022). In a final section, I discuss the implications of this explanation of Cotard delusion for the debate between one- and two factor theorists.

Interoceptive Active Inference and the Self-Model

Active inference is a theory that integrates biophysical and neurocomputational principles, but the core idea of self-modelling it entails is simple and theory-neutral. The self is a representation postulated by the brain that abstracts from, simplifies and unifies systemic functioning for regulatory purposes (Brühl, Rufer et al. 2011; Ainley, Maister et al. 2013; Seth 2013; Tsakiris and Critchley 2016; Hohwy and Michael 2017; Seth and Tsakiris 2018; Tsakiris and De Preester 2018). For example, we cannot directly change cell metabolism when energy is depleted, but we can manage fatigue by resting or drinking coffee, actions that program the innumerable interacting microprocesses required to replenish energy. The self is modelled by the mind as the entity whose energy state is changed by regulatory action. This idea generalises to higher-level, more complex forms of control over different time scales: at all levels the self is modelled as the entity whose feelings are modulated by activity and successful action consolidates that model. This self is effectively an icon the brain uses to steer the organism through the world. This icon (henceforth I will call it an avatar because the self is like an avatar used by the brain to play the game of life) is manoeuvred through bodily and affective state space by the brain as a *proxy* for the constellation of processes whose integration and regulation is necessary to maintain organismic integrity and viability (Joffily and Coricelli 2013; Limanowski and Blankenburg 2013; Velasco and Loev 2020).

The avatar vertically integrates different levels and dimensions of functioning, from basic homeostatic regulation to social and personal. Its lowest levels integrate signals of the state of the internal milieu such as blood oxygenation and electrolyte balance. The avatar integrates these signals in a process known as interoception, which produces a feeling of embodied selfhood. At the highest level of regulation, these states are felt as affective and bodily experiences belonging to *me* that are available to executive processes of memory, decision-making and inference and reported and communicated by the so-called narrative I. So as an idealization and simplification, we can say that the avatar has a 'spine' of interconnected and interacting bodily and narrative processes, each of which has a neural hub. The lowest levels of processing integrated by the avatar are interoceptive, the highest levels are narrative and conceptual and these levels are integrated by affective processing that allows us to feel the significance and value of information acquired in sensation. For this reason, the processes that produce affective experience look 'up' to higher-order conceptual and narrative processing and 'down' to basic sensorimotor and visceromotor processing. Affective experience is best thought of as resulting from the transcription of interoceptive signals by emotional processes that inform the subject of the emotional salience of the body state in context (For example raised heartbeat, sensed in interoception, is felt differently in an episode of fear or exhilaration because the emotional contexts are different).

What we can call hubs of bodily, affective and narrative self-modelling determine patterns of distributed processing across the brain according to the goals of the organism represented at different levels of complexity and abstraction. Vertically they comprise the 'spine' of the avatar, and horizontally they co-ordinate the interactions between processing systems. Once again as an idealisation and abstraction, we can say that the posterior insula is a hub of basic bodily aspects of self-modelling sensed in interoception, and the anterior insula is a hub of affective aspects of experience (Gu, Hof et al. 2013; Frot, Faillenot et al. 2014; Moayedi 2014). As a result, patterned activity across the insula implements the avatar that allows us to feel that bodily, perceptual and cognitive episodes of a life belong to the same simple unified entity: me (Craig 2009, 2010). However insula activity comprises a continuous gradient from multisensory and embodied input-integration to complex behavioural regulation as one moves along the posterior-to-anterior axis ... posterior insula exhibits mostly multi-sensory responses and is broadly connected to thalamic and primary sensory regions; the anterior insula is instead responsive to attentional (salience, response inhibition) and affective (emotion regulation and awareness) conditions and sends projections to the parietal-frontal control regions and brainstem nuclei (Allen et al. 2016a; Cerliani et al. 2012; Klein et al. 2013; Uddin 2015), with both profiles being freely mixed in the middle insula. Interoceptive predictive coding thus argues that the *insular cortex integrates low-level sensory prediction errors with interoceptive and attentional expectations to regulate affective salience and emotion* (Allen and Friston 2018).

Thus, the insula is a key system that ensures that experiences are felt to matter to me, bodily and affectively (Craig 2009). Its activity provides the foundation for the feeling of being a continuous unified self. These feelings are interpreted, reported and communicated by higher levels of narrative or conceptual self-modelling in which we explicitly represent autobiographical episodes. When the self-modelling system is functioning effectively, bodily, affective and conceptual representations of the self enable adaptive action. Importantly the idea of the hierarchical self model does not imply separate bodily affective and narrative selves. Rather, patterned activity across systems that integrate interoception, emotion and explicit autobiographical representation produces the feeling of being a persisting, unified entity that has bodily/affective and sensory/cognitive experiences.

Depersonalization Experience and the Insula: Dissociative Deaffectualisation

This role for the anterior insula helps explain why (1) anterior insula hypoactivity is associated with reduced or absent affect and (2) hypoactivity is associated with depersonalisation.

The deaffectualisation account of depersonalisation experience unifies the explanation of these phenomena. On this account, the causally responsible mechanism is spontaneous inhibition of anterior insula cortex by the ventrolateral prefrontal cortex as a dissociative response to actual or anticipated trauma (Phillips, Medford et al. 2001; Medford, Brierley et al. 2006; Medford and Critchley 2010; Medford 2012; Sierra, Medford et al. 2012; Medford, Sierra et al. 2016). The core of the account is that higher-level regulatory systems deactivate the anterior insula in order to reduce or remove a distress response in situations where the subject cannot take action to avert or avoid it. Thus Sierra:

> depersonalization represents an anxiety-triggered 'hard-wired' inhibitory response intended to ensure the preservation of adaptive behavior during situations normally associated with overwhelming and potentially disorganizing anxiety.
>
> (Sierra 2008)

The result is affective flattening or deaffectualisation while cognition, perception and the cognitive and expressive (behavioral) aspects of emotion remain intact. Thus, we find reports such as

> *It almost feels like I have died*, but no one has thought to tell me. So, I'm left living in a shell that I don't recognize any more. (Medford, Sierra et al. 2016)
>
> (my italics)

Of course, given the integrative role of the anterior insula cortex and its dense multidirectional coupling and functional connectivity, there may be no unique cause of anterior insula hypoactivity or the cause of depersonalisation experience. Dissociative deaffectualisation produced by spontaneous inhibition might be an extreme case. In other cases, depersonalisation arises over a long period typically of anxious rumination on life events felt to be inescapable. Anterior insula dysfunction could result from reduced connectivity with interoceptive afferents or lost connectivity with limbic systems that evaluate perceptual and interoceptive signals for emotional relevance. In any case, if the anterior insula cortex is hypoactive and other hubs and dimensions of self-representation, bodily, agential, sensorimotor, and narrative are intact, the result is feelings of detachment and estrangement. The reason is that the anterior insula cortex is no longer functioning to allow her to feel the significance of bodily changes evoked by activities as she engages with the world. This is perhaps why depersonalisation experience is characteristic of many psychiatric conditions (and induced by drugs such as ketamine). Because the insula is a hub, there is no single pathway to its modulation. Equally its modulation, including deactivation has widespread effects. The unifying feature is that in all cases they will be felt as changes to the quality of self-awareness with dissociated deaffectualisation an extreme case.

The second point to note about this account is that it depends essentially not just on the fact that anterior insula activity is associated with affective states, but that those states are predicted to occur in emotionally salient contexts. The subject feels depersonalised, not just because he lacks affect but because the mind *predicts* that activity such as hugging one's children will produce an affective response or that bereavement will be distressing. In the terms of the explanation, we have proposed the subject has an intact self-model that predicts affective consequences of activity. She experiences and regulates body states as hers because the posterior insula is intact, and she can narrate and conceptualise experiences because the Default Mode Network is intact, but life is no longer felt to matter to her because the affective dimension of self-modelling is absent. She feels like a marionette going through the motions.

One interesting feature of this account is that it lays the basis for a fairly straightforward 'affective' theory of depersonalisation and the Cotard delusion, in which loss of affective response produces depersonalisation (the subject feels as if she does not exist because she lacks affective response), and the Cotard delusion is an hypothesis that explains that experience. Indeed, at the dawn of the millennium, I and others proposed such a theory (Gerrans 2000). In effect such a theory is very similar to the two factor theory but proposes that the cause of depersonalisation is deaffectualisation. However Cotard and Davies point out simple loss of affect is neither necessary nor sufficient for depersonalisation or Cotard delusion. People who lose affective response do not report depersonalisation, and in some cases (more controversial; see Gerrans 2022) depersonalisation coexists with a negatively valenced experience.

Simple deaffectualisation theory is thus not adequate to the phenomena of either depersonalisation or Cotard delusion (Davies and Coltheart 2022), although I think it is on the right track. It is not just that affect is lacking in the dissociative cases but that affect signals whether and how things matter to *me* in a way that allows the me to change my experience fortunes by acting. When experiences predicted by the self-model to have affective consequences lack that 'emotional colouring' as Sierra calls it and regulatory responses fail, the subject begins to feel as though experiences do not belong to her.

The Cotard Delusion

The Cotard delusion is part of a rare psychiatric syndrome named after Jules Cotard. The Cotard delusion is sometimes described as the delusion that the subject has died, although it is better described as a delusion of inexistence (*délire de negation*). The delusion is part of a wider syndrome that includes anomalous and often spectacular and inexplicable bodily experiences. Often these experiences arise in the context of an episode of profound depression or as a reaction to trauma. There is no single or simple neural correlate or aetiology. Cotard delusion has been found in cases of affective disorders and schizophrenia, neurosyphilis, acute encephalitis, sub-dural haemorrhage, arteriovenous malformations, brain neoplasms, migraine, Parkinson's disease, semantic dementia, cerebrovascular disease and epilepsy, among others (Mendez and Ramírez-Bermúdez 2011; Ramirez Bermúdez et al. 2020; Sahoo and Josephs 2018).

The following describes a case arising in the context of anti NMDAR encephalitis. This patient was the subject of one of the recent and rare imaging studies of this disorder. I quote the description in detail because it gives a sense of the extremity of bodily experiences that are part of the syndrome.

> After claiming to be dead, Mr. A, a 19-year-old man, was referred to the National Institute of Neurology and Neurosurgery of Mexico, because of psychotic and catatonic symptoms. According to his mother, one month before admission, his appetite had diminished, he barely slept at night and, during the day, he stayed withdrawn and silent. Mr. A would complain about his body, saying that his tendons had dried up and that his organs, particularly his heart, were getting bigger. He would speak of an internal haemorrhage: all his organs had been torn apart. Mr. A began to insist that he was dead: 'I can no longer feel the blood flowing through my veins'. This assertion did not deprive him of looking for

sharp objects to cut his neck and forearms, what he tried on multiple occasions to commit suicide. Gradually, his behaviour became disorganised: he began to urinate on his clothes, refused to eat, and his verbal production diminished to mutism.

Four days after he received his fifth session of plasma exchange, his alertness improved, but psychotic symptoms remained. When asked how he felt, he answered: '*I do not have feelings because I am dead … All human beings will be dead.*' He added that he had a 'right-sided' heart and that it had stopped.

The patient was transferred to the neuropsychiatric unit. Over the following days, catatonic symptoms continued to improve (BFCRS score of 8/21), but nihilistic delusions persisted unchanged: '*I am dead, among other human beings. This is like a program where I am dead*'. The patient claimed to be a dead person among the corpses under the earthquake debris. Doctors and nurses were part of a game whose objective was to cover up his death.

(Ramirez Bermúdez, Bustamante-Gomez et al. 2020)

While it is clear that depersonalisation can be part of the Cotard syndrome, particularly in cases with a protracted progressive onset, it also seems that the syndrome is characterised by a wide network of interrelated bodily and cognitive symptoms. It also seems clear that the Cotard delusion is not essentially dissociative. Depersonalisation is often part of the Cotard syndrome, but selective suppression of affect is not a good way to characterise the precipitating experience of Cotard delusion (So Gerrans 2000 was wrong. A case of a philosopher acknowledging in print!). Not least because Cotard patients can experience extreme and fluctuating negative affect.

I suggest that the best way to explain the Cotard delusion is not in terms of depersonalisation but in terms of the underlying cognitive cause of the syndrome of which it is a part. At the neurobiological level, that cause is intractable inability of the mind to regulate basic bodily functioning. At the level of cognition, this is reflected in disintegration of the self model. It is not bodily dysregulation per se that is the essence of the Cotard delusion but the constitutive disintegration of the self model that goes along with that dysregulation. Stephan et al. have given a beautiful example of the way sustained dysregulation can corrode the self modelling process in their *dyshomeostasis* explanation of depression.

Imagine being unable to sleep properly for weeks or months. In such a case a very basic mechanism of bodily regulation essential to bodily and cognitive function is out of kilter. Such intractable insomnia can be the result of endogenously caused failure of homeostatic systems, or intractably stressful physical or social environments or, very likely, a combination. Whatever the precise pathway, when the subject cannot regulate basic biological functioning such as sleep, the consequences cascade through the control hierarchy. The first stage is at the level of interoceptive self-modelling

> the emitted control actions cannot reduce interoceptive surprise, a meta-cognitive interpretation ensues that leads to the subjective feeling of fatigue.
>
> (Stephan et al. 2016, p. 17)

At higher levels of control, the subject tries cognitive and behavioural strategies to reduce fatigue. However all strategies fail, which teaches the subject that no matter what the subject does, she cannot control her*self* at the most basic bodily level.

> an agent's experience of enduring *dyshomeostasis* signals a fundamental lack of mastery and control (over bodily states and thus survival) which may generalize, from the allostatic domain to other cognitive domains that are crucial for self-evaluation, planning and action selection.
>
> (Stephan et al. 2016, p. 17)

This is essentially a bottom-up account of the cognitive aspects of depression: thoughts of failure, worthlessness and inefficacy are consequent on basic failures of bodily self-regulation. Thus, intractable fatigue becomes apathy, misery, 'sickness behaviour', and higher-level cognition reflects this systemic failure in thoughts of failure, hopelessness and worthlessness. Stephan et al. don't describe the architecture that produces depressive symptoms as a result of dyshomeostasis, but they note that the insula is a key component of a control hierarchy that progressively re-maps interoceptive signals and integrates them with higher level forms of self-representation involved in cognitive control. The result is that on their theory, high-level metacognitive states such as depressive beliefs are a 'consequence not a cause' of lower level regulatory and self-modelling failure. Another way to put this is to say that the subject can no longer perform allostatic active inference across the hierarchy. There is no necessary bottom-up cause of depressive dyshomeostasis. Given bidirectional signalling across the hierarchy and the regulatory role of high-level self-modelling, cognitive responses to adverse or predicted adverse life events can eventually reconfigure lower-level processing. Indeed Cotard (1880) himself noted 'le malade s'accuse lui-meme'.

This model postulates a control hierarchy that links a key homeostatic process, energy regulation, to depressive symptoms. There are numerous other pathologies that can induce dyshomeostasis, including cancers, and chemotherapy and, tellingly in cases such as that of Mr A., autoimmune diseases such as encephalitis. In the latter cases the dysregulation can be even more pervasive and resistant to regulation than fatigue. This is evident in the panoply of bodily symptoms produced by NMDAR encephalitis.

In cases like the ones described by Ramirez Bermúdez and collaborators, the patient experiences a catastrophic and chaotic failure across the hierarchy of systemic regulation. In such a situation there is *no* adequate bodily self-model that predicts the consequences of regulatory action and no predictable transcription of such chaotic interoceptive states into affective experience that can serve as a regulatory proxy. Bodily and affective states can still be sensed because sensory systems are not destroyed but the self-model that integrates sensori- and visceromotor processing for regulatory purposes no longer exists. The most basic structure of self-regulation has disintegrated from the bottom up.

In another example Ramirez Bermúdez et al. describe a patient whose admission to hospital was preceded by feelings of physical and mental weakness following the Mexico City earthquake. His symptoms are an inventory of cascading dysregulation.

> headaches, insomnia, decreased appetite, irritability, auditory and visual hallucinations, delusions, and prolonged periods of mutism, and aggressive behavior toward himself and others. He also became paranoid, believing that his family wanted to harm him…
>
> fluctuating levels of consciousness with periods of psychomotor agitation, inattention, and disorientation.
>
> autonomic instability and catatonic features, including motor excitement alternating with immobility, mutism, staring, and posturing.
>
> (Ramirez Bermúdez et al. 2020)

In severe cases like NMDAR encephalitis, the mind learns that there is no viable regulatory target because experience is chaotic and unpredictable. The self, understood as the entity that sustains a predictable and regulable internal milieu, has disintegrated.

The concept of catastrophic dyshomeostasis suggests that while insula dysfunction may be common to depersonalisation experience and the Cotard delusion, the inference that the resultant experience *is the same in each case* is not licensed by that fact. Dissociative deaffectualisation is a selective phenomenon in depersonalisation that mainly affects affective regulation and response. Mr A experienced a catastrophic and pervasive disintegration of bodily and affective regulation.

Without pushing the analogy too hard, we can compare insula hypoactivity in depersonalisation and the Cotard delusion to the experience of prosopagnosia consequent on abnormal activity of the facial fusiform gyrus in different forms of prosopagnosia. (Bornstein and Kidron 1959; Barton, Davies-Thompson et al. 2021). Prosopagnosia is a disorder of face recognition explained in terms of the implementation of a neurocomputational model. We might say that depersonalisation is like associative prosopagnosia in which the subject can still represent faces and their features but has lost the sense of familiarity for that person. Most of the representational architecture of face recognition is intact but the sense of *relevance to me* is absent. In apperceptive prosopagnosia, the architecture of face recognition is severely impaired so that a subject may be unable to represent and integrate facial features at all. Her experience when seeing a face is more chaotic because the model on which face recognition depends has degraded. In apperceptive propopagnosia, it is not just that she cannot identify the face; she cannot represent it *as a face* even if she can identify features individually.

One aspect of this analogy that is useful is that face recognition is a modelling process with a complex architecture that integrates information from multiple, distributed sources. The facial fusiform gyrus is a *hub* of this integrated processing, which suggests that inability to recognise faces can take different forms and can be caused by partial of or total failure of the modelling process with multiple aetiologies depending on the interactions of different components of the system and the nature and degree of dysfunction of the facial fusiform gyrus.

So, on this analogy, depersonalisation is like associative prosopagnosia: one type of information cannot be annexed to a largely intact model. The Cotard delusion is more like apperceptive prosopagnosia in which the model has disintegrated. As a result, in the Cotard delusion, the self, *understood as the entity that unifies and integrates systemic function*, is no longer represented and felt to be present in experience.

Before comparing this account to the elegant two factor neuropsychiatric account, we need to describe that account in a little more detail.

The Two Factor Neuropsychiatric Account

The two factor account is nicely summarised in a recent paper by Coltheart and Davies.

> any (monothematic) delusional condition is initially triggered by observation of a Surprising Event (SE), *the occurrence of which is a consequence of the hypothesised First Factor, that is a neuropsychological impairment or some other abnormality*. The resulting delusional idea comes to mind as *an attempt to explain this observation*—that is, to render the event unsurprising.
>
> (Davies and Coltheart 2022, p. 436, my italics)

A version that fits this template for the Cotard delusion is an explanation in which abnormal insular function produces the experience of (inter alia) depersonalisation, in which the subject feels 'as if' she is not present in experience. This is the first factor in the genesis of the delusion. The second factor is malfunction of higher-level metacognitive systems that reconciles the content of experience with background knowledge. Due to malfunction of these systems, the subject 'endorses' or 'takes at face value' the content of depersonalisation experience and forms the belief that she does not exist. Putting things this way combines the phenomenological account of the Cotard delusion of Alexandre Billon (2016) with the cognitive neuropsychiatric account of Ramirez Bermúdez and collaborators who say:

> an interruption between the normal processing of internal and external stimuli in the IC [insular cortex] and other limbic areas could result in *abnormal subjective feeling states* (Namkung et al., 2017) that could represent a first factor for the development of nihilistic delusions described by patients with Cotard syndrome.
>
> (Ramirez Bermúdez, Bustamante-Gomez et al. 2020)

As a result, they propose a cognitive architecture that explains the relationship between insula dysfunction, depersonalisation and Cotard delusion in the diagram below.

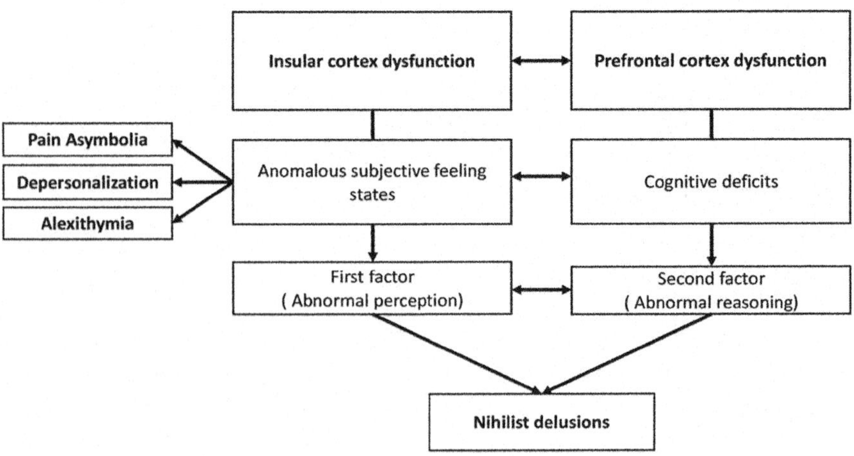

Figure 8.1 Relationship between insula dysfunction, depersonalisation and Cotard delusion.

Billon similarly explains the essence of the combined account as follows:

> Even though they are not delusional, depersonalised patients seem to display a phenomenology that is quite similar to that of Cotard patients. ... Cotard's nihilistic delusions, I argue, simply *consist in taking this altered phenomenology at face value*.
>
> (Billon 2016, p. 23)

One feature of this two factor approach emphasised by Coltheart and Davies is the relation between the precipitating anomalous experience and the delusional belief 'I have died/do not exist'. As they say, depersonalisation can plausibly prompt such a thought as an automatically generated abductive inference. The delusion is then explained in terms of *failure to override* that delusional inference. That failure derives from some sort of metacognitive deficit, a bias or deficit in rational evaluation.

A Second Factor in Cotard Delusion?

Second-factor explanations like those of Billon, Coltheart and Davies, Chatterjee and Mitra (Chatterjee and Mitra 2015) and Ramirez Bermúdez et al. agree that anomalous experience of depersonalisation is insufficient to explain the delusion. The delusion required an additional metacognitive deficit. That consists in endorsing or taking at face value the content of a depersonalisation experience. But, as with many delusions, that does not seem to be quite the case. The inability to override the delusion coexists with rational insight. Charland Verville's patient is just one of many.

> He acknowledged that his abilities to see, hear, think, remember and communicate proved that his mind must be alive: he could not explain how his mind could be alive if his brain was dead, but he was certain that this was the case.
>
> (Charland-Verville, Bruno et al. 2013)

This is not quite an 'as if' report, but it does show a degree of rational insight, as do many patients. For example:

> When I reflect on my situation, I cannot understand it at all. Either I am alive or I am not alive, but I cannot be dead as my heart beats, but I am not alive as my person has disappeared. ... I feel like not being someone and nevertheless I talk, am I stupid? *I am a body without a soul*. ... It's more complicated than the Holy Trinity.
>
> (Janet's [1928, 43] patient Laetitia, emphasis mine; quoted in Billon 2016)

In another account a patient was asked:

E: *Do you rationally think you are dead?*
P: *I do. It may not make much sense since I realize I have blood pressure when they measure it but I rationally think I am dead. (Gonçalves and Tosoni 2016, p. 35)*

Whatever the precise nature of the higher-level anomalies in the Cotard delusion, it does not seem right to say that it amounts to taking experience at face value, inability to detect inconsistency with background knowledge, or failing to understand requirements of procedural rationality.

A suggestion that preserves the insight that the anomalous experience is insufficient for delusion switches the emphasis from cognition to regulation. Epistemically the patient has intact knowledge that bodily experience and inexistence of the self are inconsistent. But that knowledge has no regulatory impact because the self-model has disintegrated; she cannot do anything to manage or modulate anomalous bodily and affective experience. In that sense she is correct to report that 'she' does not exist. Where of course 'she' refers to the experience of being regulator and regulatory target. Active inference is disabled.

I am not proposing this as a 'one-factor' account. My main purpose has been to distinguish the precipitating experience in depersonalisation and Cotard delusion. However, in the case of Mr A, the problem does *not* seem to be understanding that the delusional belief is irrational but rather the inability to take any action that could alter or remediate the experience of non-existence of the avatar. In this respect at least, the Cotard delusion is similar to dissociative deaffectualisation in that the experience produced by disrupted self-modelling is intractable and unpredictable.

Other Paths to Delusion. The Narrative Level of Self-Modelling

The self-modelling account postulates a hierarchical self-model that anchors processing across the mind through reciprocal interaction with distributed processing systems required for self-referential tasks. This suggests that there is no single pathway to damage or disintegration of the self-model. Extreme dyshomeostasis is a bottom-up phenomenon, but in principle the self-model could be affected at any level with cascading vertical and horizontal effects. This explains the role of damage to the Default Mode Network (DMN), hub of the narrative level of self-modelling observed in other cases of Cotard delusion.

A role for the DMN was identified in a PET study by Charland Verville et al. of a man referred to psychiatric services after an electrocution attempt. This man had almost complete atrophy of the default mode network (Charland-Verville, Bruno et al. 2013; Chatterjee and Mitra 2015). Ramirez Bermúdez in their imaging studies noted hypoactivity of the DMN and its role in 'integrating information from multiple sources, including autobiographical memory and interoceptive processes, suggesting an active role of the DMN in the neural construction of the self' (Ramirez Bermúdez, Bustamante-Gomez et al. 2020). The best way to conceptualise the role of the DMN is at the top level of the self-modelling hierarchy. It assembles and associates information necessary for the subject to experience herself in episodes of autobiographical thought. It communicates with hubs of emotional processing and insular circuitry to allow explicit autobiographical representations to be felt as affectively salient, providing the material for autobiographical narrative.

The DMN is connected to both hubs of emotional processing and to the insula cortex. On some views it is a substrate of the narrative 'I'.

As Davey et al put it:

> The DMN therefore coordinates a sense of self that spans cognitive abstractions about the self with a more grounded awareness of the state of the body.
>
> (Davey and Harrison 2018)

This is consistent with the role I described for the DMN as a hub of higher-level narrative self modelling that reciprocally modulates affective and interoceptive self modelling.

This role for the DMN reflects its activation in a wide variety of high-level self-referential activities such as rumination, episodic memory, planning, imagination, dreaming. It is an integrative hub that allows the subject to experience affectively inflected experiences as episodes in the life of a temporally extended and unified self. As such, if the default network is damaged or disconnected from the more basic forms of bodily/affective selfhood, then the ability to represent the self as an embodied persisting entity that sustains an autobiography will be compromised.

Conclusion

It is worth recalling at this point the fundamental idea behind the active inference account of self-modelling. Namely, the mind models the self as the entity whose boundaries are maintained and internal states and structures stabilised in the face of entropic forces acting on living systems (Corcoran and Hohwy 2017; Kirchhoff, Parr et al. 2018; van Es 2021). This modelling process is hierarchical, recruiting cognitive processes at levels appropriate to the regulatory tasks. A crucial part of the story is that the self is an *avatar* manoeuvred through bodily and affective state space by the brain as a *proxy* for the constellation of processes whose integration and regulation is necessary to resist entropy. In the normal case the narrative 'I' is subtended by the integrated hierarchy of bodily and affective processes and regulatory models whose trajectory it racks, predicts, interprets and communicates.

On this view, cascading bottom-up damage to the hierarchical self-model will effectively hollow it out. The narrative I becomes disembodied, and if the DMN is also disabled or impaired, then the ability to represent a coherent autobiographical trajectory is also lost. Jean, a Cotard patient studied by Young and Leafhead, described herself as 'just a voice and if that goes I won't be anything. … [I]f my voice goes I will be lost and I won't know where I have gone' (Young and Leafhead 1996).

In Cotard syndrome, the panoply of associated bodily and cognitive symptoms, rotting, translucency, distortion, disappearance, the sense that the mind and person herself are disappearing combined with the aetiologies of depression, trauma or low-level malfunction and psychosis seem to differentiate the experience from depersonalisation. The experience of depersonalisation does seem to be essentially dissociative and relatively circumscribed. Insula hypoactivity in this case impairs the ability to self-model affective experience while sparing (to a greater or lesser degree) self-modelling of other bodily and cognitive processes. At the same time, the self-modelling account is also consistent with the idea that depersonalisation experience could overlap with other bodily and interoceptive dysfunctions precisely because the insula cortex, like other components of the model, is an integrative hub, not a discrete module with a single function (Moayedi 2014; Betti and Aglioti 2016; Pessoa 2017).

References

Ainley, V., et al. (2013). "More of myself: Manipulating interoceptive awareness by heightened attention to bodily and narrative aspects of the self." *Consciousness and Cognition* **22**(4): 1231–1238.

Allen, M. (2020). "Unravelling the neurobiology of interoceptive inference." *Trends in Cognitive Sciences* **24**(4): 265–266.

Allen, M. and K. J. Friston (2018). "From cognitivism to autopoiesis: Towards a computational framework for the embodied mind." *Synthese* **195**(6): 2459–2482.

Barrett, L. F., et al. (2016). "An active inference theory of allostasis and interoception in depression." *Philosophical Transactions of the Royal Society B* **371** (1708): 20160011.

Barrett, L. F. and W. K. Simmons (2015). "Interoceptive predictions in the brain." *Nature Reviews Neuroscience* **16**(7): 419–429.

Barton, J. J. S., et al. (2021). "Prosopagnosia and disorders of face processing." *Handbook of Clinical Neurology* **178**: 175–193.

Betti, V. and S. M. Aglioti (2016). "Dynamic construction of the neural networks underpinning empathy for pain." *Neuroscience & Biobehavioral Reviews* **63**: 191–206.

Billon, A. (2016). "Making sense of the Cotard syndrome: Insights from the study of depersonalisation." *Mind & Language* **31**(3): 356–391.

Bornstein, B. and D. P. Kidron (1959). "Prosopagnosia." *Journal of Neurology, Neurosurgery, and Psychiatry* **22**(2): 124–131.

Brühl, A. B., M. Rufer, A. Delsignore, T. Kaffenberger, L. Jäncke, and U. Herwig (2011). "Neural correlates of altered general emotion processing in social anxiety disorder." *Brain Research* **1378**: 72–83.

Cauda, F., et al. (2011). "Functional connectivity of the insula in the resting brain." *NeuroImage* **55**(1): 8–23.

Cerliani, L., et al. (2012). "Probabilistic tractography recovers a rostrocaudal trajectory of connectivity variability in the human insular cortex." *Human Brain Mapping* **33**(9): 2005–2034.

Charland-Verville, V., et al. (2013). "Brain dead yet mind alive: A positron emission tomography case study of brain metabolism in Cotard's syndrome." *Cortex* **49**(7): 1997–1999.

Chatterjee, S. S. and S. Mitra (2015). ""I do not exist"—Cotard syndrome in insular cortex atrophy." *Biological Psychiatry* **77**(11): e52–e53.

Corcoran, A. W. and J. Hohwy (2017). "Allostasis, interoception, and the free energy principle: Feeling our way forward."

Corcoran, A. W., et al. (2020). "From allostatic agents to counterfactual cognisers: Active inference, biological regulation, and the origins of cognition." *Biology and Philosophy* **35**(3): 1–45.

Cotard, J. (1891). *Études sur les maladies cérébrales et mentales*. J-B. Baillère. available at http://gallica.bnf.fr.

Craig, A. (2009a). "Emotional moments across time: A possible neural basis for time perception in the anterior insula." *Philosophical Transactions: Biological Sciences* **364**: 1933–1942.

Craig, A. D. (2009b). "How do you feel—now? the anterior insula and human awareness." *Nature Reviews Neuroscience* **10**(1): 59–70.

Craig, A. D. (2010). "The sentient self." *Brain Structure and Function* **214**: 563–577.

Davey, C. G. and B. J. Harrison (2018). "The brain's center of gravity: How the default mode network helps us to understand the self." *World Psychiatry* **17**(3): 278.

Davies, M. and M. Coltheart (2022). "Cotard delusion, emotional experience and depersonalisation." *Cognitive Neuropsychiatry* **27**(6): 430–446.

Deane, G., et al. (2020). "Losing ourselves: Active inference, depersonalization and meditation." *Frontiers in Psychology* **11**: 2893.

Friston, K., et al. (2011). "Action understanding and active inference." *Biological Cybernetics* **104**(1–2): 137–160.

Frot, M., et al. (2014). "Processing of nociceptive input from posterior to anterior insula in humans." *Human Brain Mapping* **35**(11): 5486–5499.

Gerrans, P. (2000). "Refining the explanation of Cotard's delusion." *Mind & Language* **15**(1): 111–122.

Gerrans, P. (2019). "Depersonalization disorder, affective processing and predictive coding." *Review of Philosophy and Psychology* **10**(2): 401–418.

Gerrans, P. (2020). "Pain asymbolia as depersonalization for pain experience. An interoceptive active inference account." *Frontiers in Psychology* **11**.

Gerrans, P. (2022). "A vessel without a pilot: Bodily and affective experience in the Cotard delusion of inexistence." *Mind & Language*. https://doi.org/10.1111/mila.12441

Gerrans, P. and R. J. Murray (2020). "Interoceptive active inference and self-representation in social anxiety disorder (SAD): Exploring the neurocognitive traits of the SAD self." *Neuroscience of Consciousness*.

Gonçalves, L. M. and A. Tosoni (2016). "Sudden onset of Cotard's syndrome as a clinical sign of brain tumor." *Archives of Clinical Psychiatry* (São Paulo) **43**: 35–36.

Gu, X., P. R. Hof, K. J. Friston, and J. Fan (2013). "Anterior insular cortex and emotional awareness." *Journal of Comparative Neurology* **521**(15): 3371–3388.

Hohwy, J. and J. Michael (2017). "Why Should Any Body Have a Self?" In F. De Vignemont and A. J. T. Alsmith (Eds.), *The Subject's Matter: Self-Consciousness and the Body* (pp. 363–391). Cambridge, MA: MIT Press.

Huebner, B. and J. Schulkin (2022). *Biological Cognition*. Cambridge: Cambridge University Press.

Joffily, M. and G. Coricelli (2013). "Emotional valence and the free-energy principle." *PLoS Computational Biology* **9**(6): e1003094.

Kirchhoff, M., et al. (2018). "The Markov blankets of life: Autonomy, active inference and the free energy principle." *Journal of the Royal Society Interface* **15**(138): 20170792.

Klein, T. A., M. Ullsperger, and C. Danielmeier (2013). "Error awareness and the insula: links to neurological and psychiatric diseases." *Frontiers in Human Neuroscience* **7**: 14.

Limanowski, J. and F. Blankenburg (2013). "Minimal self-models and the free energy principle." *Frontiers in Human Neuroscience* **7**: 547.

Medford, N. (2012). "Emotion and the unreal self: Depersonalization disorder and de-affectualization." *Emotion Review* **4**(2): 139–144.

Medford, N., et al. (2006). "Emotional memory in depersonalization disorder: A functional MRI study." *Psychiatry Research: Neuroimaging* **148**(2): 93–102.

Medford, N. and H. D. Critchley (2010). "Conjoint activity of anterior insular and anterior cingulate cortex: Awareness and response." *Brain Structure and Function* **214**(5–6): 535–549.

Medford, N., et al. (2016). "Emotional experience and awareness of self: Functional MRI studies of depersonalization disorder." *Frontiers in Psychology* **7**: 432.

Mendez, Mario F. and Jesús Ramírez-Bermúdez (2011). "Cotard syndrome in semantic dementia." *Psychosomatics* **52**(6): 571.

Moayedi, M. (2014). "All roads lead to the insula." *Pain* **155**(10): 1920–1921.

Parr, T. and K. J. Friston (2017). "Uncertainty, epistemics and active inference." *Journal of the Royal Society Interface* **14**(136): 20170376.

Parr, T., G. Pezzulo, and K. J. Friston (2022). *Active Inference: The Free Energy Principle in Mind, Brain, and Behavior*. Cambridge, MA: MIT Press.

Paulus, M. P. and M. B. Stein (2010). "Interoception in anxiety and depression." *Brain Structure and Function* **214**(5–6): 451–463.

Pessoa, L. (2017). "A network model of the emotional brain." *Trends in Cognitive Sciences* **21**(5): 357–371.

Pezzulo, G., et al. (2015). "Active inference, homeostatic regulation and adaptive behavioural control." *Progress in Neurobiology* **134**: 17–35.

Phillips, M. L., et al. (2001). "Depersonalization disorder: Thinking without feeling." *Psychiatry Research: Neuroimaging* **108**(3): 145–160.

Ramirez Bermúdez, J., et al. (2020). "Cotard syndrome in anti-NMDAR encephalitis: Two patients and insights from molecular imaging." *Neurocase*: 1–8.

Restrepo-Martínez, M., et al. (2019). "FDG-PET in Cotard syndrome before and after treatment: Can functional brain imaging support a two-factor hypothesis of nihilistic delusions?" *Cognitive Neuropsychiatry* **24**(6): 470–480.

Sahoo, A. and K. A. Josephs (2018). "A neuropsychiatric analysis of the Cotard delusion." *The Journal of Neuropsychiatry and Clinical Neurosciences* **30**(1): 58–65.

Seth, A. K. (2013). "Interoceptive inference, emotion, and the embodied self." *Trends in Cognitive Sciences* **17**(11): 565–573.

Seth, A. K. and K. J. Friston (2016). "Active interoceptive inference and the emotional brain." *Philosophical Transactions of the Royal Society, B: Biological Sciences* **371**(1708): 20160007.

Seth, A. K. and M. Tsakiris (2018). "Being a beast machine: The somatic basis of selfhood." *Trends in Cognitive Sciences* **22**(11): 969–981.

Sierra, M. (2008). "Depersonalization disorder: Pharmacological approaches." *Expert Review of Neurotherapeutics* **8**(1): 19–26.

Sierra, M., et al. (2012). "Depersonalization disorder and anxiety: A special relationship?" *Psychiatry Research* **197**(1): 123–127.

Starr, C. J., et al. (2009). "Roles of the insular cortex in the modulation of pain: Insights from brain lesions." *Journal of Neuroscience* **29**(9): 2684–2694.

Stephan, K. E., et al. (2016). "Allostatic self-efficacy: A metacognitive theory of dyshomeostasis-induced fatigue and depression." *Frontiers in Human Neuroscience* **10**: 550.

Terasawa, Y., et al. (2013). "Anterior insular cortex mediates bodily sensibility and social anxiety." *Social Cognitive and Affective Neuroscience* **8**(3): 259–266.

Tsakiris, M. and H. Critchley (2016). "Interoception beyond homeostasis: Affect, cognition and mental health." *The Royal Society B: Biological Sciences* **371** (1708): 20160002.

Tsakiris, M. and H. De Preester (2018). *The Interoceptive Mind: From Homeostasis to Awareness*.Oxford: Oxford University Press.

Uddin, L. Q., J. S. Nomi, B. Hébert-Seropian, J. Ghaziri, and O. Boucher (2017). "Structure and function of the human insula." *Journal of Clinical Neurophysiology: Official Publication of the American Electroencephalographic Society* **34**(4): 300.

van Es, T. (2021). "Living models or life modelled? On the use of models in the free energy principle." *Adaptive Behavior* **29**(3): 315–329.

Velasco, P. F. and S. Loev (2020). "Affective experience in the predictive mind: A review and new integrative account." *Synthese* **198**(11): 10847–10882.

Von Mohr, M. and A. Fotopoulou (2018). "Of Interoception: Active and Social Inference of Pain and Pleasure on." In *The Interoceptive Mind: From Homeostasis to Awareness*: 102.

Young, A. W. and K. M. Leafhead (1996). "Betwixt Life and Death: Case Studies of the Cotard Delusion." In *Method in Madness: Case Studies in Cognitive Neuropsychiatry*: 147–171.

Part III

The Normative Framework of Delusion

9 From Abnormal Time-Space Experience to Delusions

Spatiotemporal Psychopathology

Filipe Arantes-Gonçalves and Georg Northoff

Introduction

Delusions are complex psychopathological symptoms where subjects attribute internally oriented thought contents to the external world. Specifically, their self generates thought contents that are solely based on their internal generation by the self itself, irrespective and independent of the external reality in the world. Unlike in healthy subjects, who can demarcate the boundaries of internally and externally generated thoughts, schizophrenia subjects remain unable to do so. They instead project the internally generated thought contents upon the external reality such that the former are taken for the latter itself – this results in what psychiatrists call delusions.

There are numerous investigations of delusions including biological, phenomenological and psychological. We here focus on the phenomenological aspect, that is the experience. Specifically, we focus on showing delusions are generated by a more basic disturbance of time-space experience. For that, we go back to an earlier phenomenological psychiatrist, Eugen Minkowski, whose view of schizophrenia as loss of vital contact with reality serves as template for the present view of delusions as a primary spatiotemporal disorder entailing what we described as Spatiotemporal Psychopathology [1–4]. In that vein, we also introduce an abbreviated version of our recently introduced Scale for Time-Space Experience in Psychosis (STEP) [5] for a more clinical routine use.

Loss of Vital Contact with Reality – Going Back to Minkowski

The concept of *schizophrenic autism* was proposed by the French psychiatrist Eugène Minkowski [6], who claimed that a patient with such a condition actively opposes (or acts in contradiction with) the ongoing dynamics of the corresponding environment. This manifests as emptiness, personality disaggregation and as static or immobilized experience of space and

DOI: 10.4324/9781003288992-13

time [7]. In other words, a patient with schizophrenic autism is not oriented towards social communication [7]. According to Minkowski, *schizophrenic autism* is characterized by the following five main features:

1. '*Loss of vital contact with reality*'. This describes the loss of motivation, curiosity, investment, and engagement into the environment. Instead of attuning to or synchronizing with the dynamics of the external environment, autistic subjects remain static. In other words, there is a static rather than dynamic experience of space and time of the environment including the own subject or self as part of it [7].
2. Minkowski conceives this static experience as the most important characteristic of autism in psychosis as the so-called *trouble générateur*, a French expression meaning 'generative disturbance' or 'generative disorder', which aimed at pointing out a sort of formal-structural complex, a basic disturbance, analogous to the physiological substrate of symptoms in somatic diseases [24]. Put simply, the so-called *trouble générateur* as basic disturbance was intended to meaningfully present the various symptoms of schizophrenia in an interconnected, interdependent and comprehensive way [8], lending homogeneity to an, otherwise, quite heterogenous condition [7].
3. *Rich and poor autism. Rich autism* is characterized by predominant fantasies and daydreaming consisting of an imaginary world with strong affective contents [7]; it literally resembles the original description by Bleuler, in which there is a compensatory predominance of fantasy and internal affects over reality. By contrast, in *poor autism*, not even an inner rich mental life apparently exists; instead, there is a loss of '*vital contact with reality*' both at the internal (mental life or the self) and the external environmental levels [9]. This may be manifested in the experience of loss of 'I' or 'me', which is replaced, for instance, by a third-person conversation. In other words, whereas in *rich autism* there is still an attempt of the healthy part of a given personality to counteract and compensate for the *trouble générateur*, in *poor autism* the personality emptiness predominates with no attempts of any compensatory strategy.
4. *Morbid rationalism*. This refers to a predominance of aberrant cognitive functioning over the emotional one. In other words, there is an overt predominance of an aberrant logical and irrational functioning over any emotional and feeling involvement. A key example here is the so-called *morbid geometrism* which corresponds to a predominance of spatial and numerical aspects of thought and life experiences [7].
5. *Abnormal time-space experience*: It is noteworthy to point out again that, according to Minkowski, the *trouble générateur* is closely related to an abnormal experience of space and time [10].(In particular, the

abnormal experience of time can be compared to a situation in which there is no future in one's own mind [11] and consequently, there is a lack of subjective experience of life and reality because 'It is only through the future that the self affirms itself as a living being'). This lack of dynamics in the experience of time leads to a predominance of static and irrational elements over the dynamic ones [10]. Ultimately, this speaks to the lack of a so-called *élan vital*, a French expression, not easily translatable, that illustrates the normal orientation towards the future of a living human [8, 10]. In short, the combination of the aforementioned features leads to implausibility of sharing experiences of space and time between the self and the others [12].

Self World Experience in Schizophrenia

Minkowski described the loss of vital contact with reality as the basic disturbance of schizophrenia. This means that they experience the world in a different way – this is further specified in current phenomenological psychopathology by the assumption of an unstable and disordered self-world structure [12–14]. This disorder or structural instability of the self-world structure provides the generative disorder, the '*trouble générateur*', that, symptomatically, is manifested in autism, and frames and organizes all subsequent changes and symptoms:

> We have previously proposed that the essential feature of schizophrenia spectrum disorders is a disturbance of the core self in its immediate relation to the world. It is important to emphasize that we are not talking about a lack or a deficit (as in 'too much or too little') but rather of an instability or dis-order. This basic disturbance of self-world relation is the generative component in the Gestalt of autism, which 'appears nowhere else in this particular fashion' and which imbues schizophrenia with an air of un-understandability [12, 13].

Due to the instability or dis-order of the self-world structure, its constituent elements, space and time as well as causality and non-contradiction, become questionable and ultimately disrupted if not dissolved in the experience of schizophrenic patients. This isolates them from the world resulting in a solipsistic or autistic attitude: 'This basic self-world structure is disturbed in schizophrenia spectrum disorders, i.e., it is constantly challenged, unstable, and oscillating, resulting in alarming and alienating anomalous self-experiences (also termed 'self-disorders'), typically occurring already in childhood or early adolescence. What is important to emphasize at this point is that the self-disorders, reflecting the unstable basic self-world structure, destabilize the natural ontological attitude and may throw the patient into a new ontological-existential perspective, an often solipsistic framework, no longer ruled by the 'natural' certitudes concerning space, time, causality, and noncontradiction' [15].

Time-Space versus Self-World – Who Is Primary and More Basic?

We can see here a slight tension or ambiguity concerning the role of time-space experience. The current phenomenological proponents seem to imply that the abnormal time-space experience is a consequence of an unstable and disordered self-world structure. In short, self-world structure is primary, time-space experience is secondary. That seems to stand counter to Minkowski himself, though. His assumption of a primary loss of vital contact with reality, for example, the world, is based on and conceived as a consequence of the loss of especially dynamics in the experience of time and space. Put briefly, time-space experience is primary while relation to the world is here a secondary consequence resulting from the former.

Is time-space experience primary, as implied by Minkowski, or secondary to an abnormal self-world structure, as entailed by current phenomenology? This depends on how one conceives the concept of 'structure' in self-world structure itself. If one conceives that structure in primarily temporal and spatial terms, the relation of the self to the world is based on the world's own constitution of time and space and how that, in turn, establishes or constitutes relation to the person and thereby its self. Following Minkowski, the constitution of this spatiotemporal relation of self and world is disrupted in schizophrenia leading to the loss of vital contact of the self with reality, for example, the world.

Alternatively, one may conceive the concept of structure in self-world structure independent and prior to the one of time-space. In that case, time-space are no longer foundational and constitutive for the self-world structure as it is the case in Minkowski. Rather than constituting the relation of self and world, for example, their self-world structure, time-space are now a manifestation of the former rather than its constitutional basis or foundation. The self-world structure is consequently primary while time-space experience remains secondary to that.

Which view holds? Based on ontological considerations, we assume that the existence and reality of the world is primary to the one of the self, including the self-world structure [3]. The world as whole constitutes the self as its part and thereby the latter's relation to the former, the self-world structure. How does the world constitute the self including its self-world structure? This is the moment where time-space come in. Presupposing a Spatiotemporal ontology with time-space as the most basic constituents of existence and reality in the world [3], time-space may be key in constituting the self, including its relation to the world, the self-world structure [16].

Taken such ontological view, time-space must be considered the most basic and fundamental constituents of the self-world structure with the latter being secondary as consequence of the former's constitutional processes. The experience of time-space may then offer insight into these basic and foundational constitutive process of the self itself, including its self-world structure. The experience of time-space is consequently more basic and thus primary to the experience of self, world and body which result as consequence of the former. Changes in time-space experience consequently resonate in abnormal experience of self, world and body. This is the view presupposed in the remainder of this chapter.

Phenomenological Psychopathology of Time and Space Experience in Schizophrenia

Phenomenology is about the experience of time in first-person perspective as distinguished from its psychological investigation in third-person perspective. This also shifts the focus to the structure and organization of experience in time consciousness. Following Minkowski, one core feature of schizophrenia is the experience of a disrupted flow of time: time no longer flows in consciousness but instead is frozen and immobilized in experience. The schizophrenic patient no longer experiences a continuous stream of time in her/his consciousness; the 'stream of consciousness' is disrupted. Relying on the philosopher Henri Bergson, Minkowski says that time consciousness lacks the '*élan vital*'.

Roughly, the concept of *élan vital* refers to a life force which, as we say here, may be better characterized as dynamic. Dynamic describes the continuous change from time point to time point, thus connecting them all with each other. Taken in that sense, dynamic as continuous change is key for life and vitality to exist; if, in contrast, dynamic is replaced by static, vitality and ultimately life itself are lost.

Specifically, due to their lacking dynamic, they remain unable to temporally synchronize with the ongoing change, that is, the dynamic of the environmental inputs. Instead of temporal synchronization with their present environmental context, that is, 'synchronism' [10], they show desynchronization and consecutively lack attunement – Minkowski speaks of a 'loss of vital contact with reality'. This may be re-formulated analogously as 'loss of dynamic contact with ongoing dynamic reality' leading to a loss of resonance or loss of 'sharing a rhythm' [17] with others and the social-environmental context [18]. The patient is 'in contradiction with the flow and dynamism of life' [7].

Minkowski also highlights two phenomenological features of explicit time. This includes what he describes as 'morbid rationalism' [6]. Due to the fact that schizophrenics lose their dynamic of time on the implicit level, they aim at reconstructing time on the explicit level [17]; this leads to excessive recruitment of cognitive facilities with hyper-reflexiveness and strong rational formalization of both inner and outer dynamic, including their own inner mental features and the outer environmental events.

Yet another more explicit feature highlighted by Minkowski is the experience of the abnormal 'spatialization of time experience'. Time is 'chopped up' in different discrete elements that, standing side by side, appear and are experienced at distinct locations in space, which the schizophrenic patient remains unable to connect and integrate. While the phenomenological focus has always been more on time experience, there is clear support for abnormal space experience in schizophrenia.

Stanghellini et al. [19] conducted a systematic study on space experience in schizophrenia. Conducting a semi-quantitative study, they observe that their subjective or personal space is experienced (i) as strange and unfamiliar; (ii) as being intruded or invaded; (iii) relation to the environmental space with distances and locations is distorted; (iv) things in space are altered in their dimensions like colour, shape, and so forth; and (v) itemization and abnormal perceptual salience of events and objects in the environment.

How are time and space experience connected? Temporal segmentation often goes along with what we describe as 'temporal spatialization', the transformation of time segments into more or less corresponding space segments (see above). This is supported by observations that past and future are associated with distinct spatial characterizations: past is 'located' on the left and upper while future is more located on the right and lower when doing schematic drawings [20]. Temporal segments are thus spatially located.

Given the close correspondence of temporal segmentation and its spatialization, one would expect that deficits in the former lead to changes in the latter. That is well fleshed out by Minkowski, who describes an abnormal spatialization of both the own thoughts and self as well as the environmental events and objects (see above): the loss of the dynamic of time including increased temporal segmentation leads to abnormal segmentation of space which, as their necessary condition [21], affects experience of the spatial location of both self and environment. Hence abnormal increase in segmentation may be shared by both time and space perception/experience of schizophrenia, which is in line with the assumption of 'itemization' as their shared feature [21]. I therefore assume that abnormal temporal segmentation in schizophrenia is manifest in increased temporal and spatial itemization.

Scale for Time-Space Experience in Psychosis (STEP) – Introduction of Short Version for Clinical Purposes

While qualitative [23] and semiqualitative [19, 21, 22] investigations of time-space experience have been conducted, a quantitative scale for time-space experience in psychosis is lacking so far. We therefore developed such scale which we recently introduced [5]. Roughly, the scale for time-space experience in psychosis (STEP) includes 12 items for time experience and 12 items for space experience as based on previous phenomenological studies. The ratings are based on an extensive psychopathological interview of the patients' experience with specific questions. The scale was probed in a sample of 10 schizophrenia subjects, 10 affective patients and 10 healthy controls. The clinical validity has shown that several items well distinguished the schizophrenia from the affective patients. Moreover, significant correlation with several psychopathological measures like the Positive and Negative Syndrome Scale (PANSS) and Ego pathology inventory was demonstrated [5].

Given that the STEP in its current version requires an extensive interview, we here present a shorter version based on rich clinical descriptions derived from in-depth qualitative interviews (particularly in schizophrenia patients). Moreover, we focused on those items that showed the highest discrimination between schizophrenia and affective psychosis in our first investigation. This includes about 8 items for the time experience while 6 items are included in the space experience. As per our original sample, these items showed the highest discrimination between schizophrenia and affective patients.

In our earlier study, we demonstrated that STEP can help differentiate patients with schizophrenia spectrum disorders from patients with predominant affective symptoms. Finally, we have found an association of STEP scores with the presence and severity of psychopathological symptoms. Taken together, our preliminary findings show that STEP might be a useful measure for the assessment of schizophrenia spectrum disorders.

Regarding the experience of time in schizophrenia, it is noteworthy to point out that the items differentiating patients belonging to the schizophrenia spectrum disorders group from the other two groups were items 3, 5, 7, 8 and 9 of the STEP time subscale. Interestingly, these items correspond to the Minkowski's original description of schizophrenic autism.

Regarding the experience of space in schizophrenia, our results show that the best single items to characterize patients with predominant psychotic symptoms were items 2, 4, 7, 12, 13 and 14 of the STEP space subscale. These results are also in line with a recent study by Stanghellini et al. [19]. In particular, item 7 may resemble the experience of 'centrality/invasiveness of the peri-personal space' [19]. Interestingly, these authors pointed out that patients with schizophrenia need a wider interpersonal space while in social interaction [19]. Moreover, item 13 may correspond to 'itemization and perceptive salience', whereas item 14 may resemble 'alteration of quality of the environment', as proposed by the same authors [19]. Moreover, items 2, 4 and 12 of the STEP space subscale seem to be related to body disturbance, perceived as an 'inner space' predisposing to space disturbances [19].

Item	Past Time Experience	Present Time Experience	Time Speed Desistegration	Time Irregularity/Imprecision	Affective Consequences of Time Desisntegration	Cognitive and Social Consequences of Time Deisntegration	Future experienced as threatening	Mental Time Travelling
Description in the Scale	There is a disconnection between past and present/future due to excess of traumatic memories or even the feeling of past as non-existing.	Present is experienced with difficulties of sharing a normal and active life with or even with significant passivity.	Time speed is experienced as slower and faster simultaneously.	Time is experinced as fragmented, with disconnectivity in its synthesis. This may manifest as time being felt as a series of photographs, snapshops or even like a zigue-zague.	Due to subjective experience of time fragmentation there are emotional consequences derived from it. Emotional time becomes also somewhat fragmented with feelings of both positive and negative valence simultaneously.	Due to the subjective experience of temporal fragmentation there is conscious awareness that the former has important implications in the ability to shynchronize with other people.	Future is experienced as a series of premonitions where sometimes something threatening is about to happen and other times future is felt as indifferent or even non existing.	Patients may feel difficulties in mental time traveling between past, present and future. This may manifest as feelings of life being restricted or stuck in the present.
Related Reference	Vogel DHV, Beecker T, Haidl T, Kupke C, Heinze M. Vogeley K, et al. Disturbed time experience during and after psychosis. Schizophr Res: Cogn. 2019 Mar; 21; 17: 2-9.	Vogel DHV, Beecker T, Haidl T, Kupke C, Heinze M. Vogeley K, et al. Disturbed time experience during and after psychosis. Schizophr Res: Cogn. 2019 Mar; 21; 17: 2-9.	Rich clinical description based on in-depth qualitative interview	Stanghellini, G et al. Psychopathology of lived time: abnormal time experience in persons with schizophrenia. Schizophrenia Bulletin. 2016. 42 (1): 45-55. https://doi.org/10.1093/schbul/sbv052	Rich clinical description based on in-depth qualitative interview	Rich clinical description based on in-depth qualitative interview	Stanghellini, G et al. Psychopathology of lived time: abnormal time experience in persons with schizophrenia. Schizophrenia Bulletin. 2016. 42 (1): 45-55. https://doi.org/10.1093/schbul/sbv052	Parnas et al. Examination of Anomalous Self Experience (EASE). Psychopathology; 2005. 38: 236-258. https://doi.org/10.1159/000088441

Figure 9.1 Time subscale-Short clinically oriented version of 'Space and Time Experience in Psychosis'-(STEP).

Item	Body Discoordination	Body Vitality	Detachment from other people	Body Identity	External Space experienced as overwhelming	Spatial Disorientation
Description in the Scale	The bodily actions are not syncronized and constituted as a whole, but rather pieced together as sucessions of singular, fragmented movements with rigid, angular and slow features.	A pervasive or frequently recurrent sense of inexplicable mental or physical fatigue, dampening of immediate aliveness, diminished energy, spontaneity, "elán".	Patients may feel detached from other people. This may manifest as a sense of remoteness from other people.	It may include perception of dimishment or constriction of single body parts or the experience of body parts or the whole body becoming thiner, shorter, enlarged, being pressed down or dimished. Also the body parts might be experienced as strange, alien, lifeless, isolated, separated from each other, dislocated or not existing.	Patients feel the external space as too much overstimulating with a lot of details and too much overwhelming. They feel confused and desorientated because they seem to experience sensorial bombardment. Patients experience stimuli coming from everywhere at the same time.	Though in a familiar or comprehensive location, subjects feel completely lost or disorientated. Spatial perspetives become misleading. These experiences are accompanyied by subjective sates of disorientation and confusion.
Related Reference	Hirjack, D. Breyer, T.Thomann, TA. Fuchs, T. Disturbance of Intentionality: a phenomenological study of Body-Affecting First-Rank Symptoms in Schizophrenia. PloS. 8(9): e73662. https://doi.org/10.1371/journal.pone.0073662	Parnas et al. Examination of Anomalous Self Experience (EASE). Psychopathology; 2005. 38: 236-258. https://doi.org/10.1159/000088441	Sass et al. Examination of Anomalous World Experience (EAWE). Psychopathology. 50 (1): 10-54.	Parnas et al. Examination of Anomalous Self Experience (EASE). Psychopathology; 2005. 38: 236-258. https://doi.org/10.1159/000088441	Stanghellini, G et al. Abnormal space experience in persons with schizophrenia: an empirical qualitative study. Schizophrenia Bulletin. 2020; 46 (3): 530-539. https://doi.org/10.1093/schbul/sbz107	Stanghellini, G et al. Abnormal space experience in persons with schizophrenia: an empirical qualitative study. Schizophrenia Bulletin. 2020; 46 (3): 530-539. https://doi.org/10.1093/schbul/sbz107

Figure 9.2 Space subscale-Short clinically-oriented version of 'Space and Time Experience in Psychosis'-(STEP).

Positive Symptoms and Delusions: 'Phenomenological Compensation' of an Abnormal Time-Space Experience of the World including Its Self-World Relation

We discussed time-space experience as basic and foundational for an abnormal self-world structure. How does this lead to the typical psychopathological symptoms like delusions? A brief generative account shall be given in the following.

The schizophrenic subjects can consequently perceive no longer any difference between different events in the external environment nor a difference of the latter to their own ongoing internal mental or cognitive events, that is, their self. They subsequently confuse their internal self with the external environment (and vice versa) as it is typical in symptoms like auditory hallucination, delusions, thought disorder, and ego- and passivity disturbances. The loss of object relation carries major psychopathological implications. If one can no longer perceive externally oriented contents in a synchronized and integrated way, one's perception turns inwards to internally oriented contents like delusions and hallucinations: these are the internal substitutes of the missing external perceptual contents the schizophrenic patients assume to be out there in the external world.

In phenomenological terms, these are conceived as secondary, reactive or even compensatory psychopathological mechanisms to cover up for the schizophrenic autism. These are regarded by Minkowski as attempts of 'phenomenological compensation' (Minkowski/Urfer-Parnas). Their main goal is to achieve, through the healthy part of the personality, a new balance between schizophrenic fragmentation and autism, from one side, and the (spatiotemporal) dynamic factors and *élan vital*, from the other.

Although they try to avoid even more schizophrenic autism and fragmentation, they are always shaped by the *trouble générateur* (fundamental disturbance in the schizophrenic process). That is why positive symptoms are most of the times characterized by lack of pragmatic value, sterility and immobility. In clinical practice, it is easily recognizable that these are often triggered by emotionally relevant stimuli. However, even guided by these affective tones, positive symptoms are not dynamically rooted in a meaningful context. By contrast, they seem to have an eccentric and detached way of reconnecting with reality. And that is precisely where it becomes evident the intrinsic psychopathological mechanism of 'phenomenological compensation' between the *trouble générateur* and the positive symptoms.

Finally, Minkowski distinguishes between two types of 'phenomenological compensation':

1. in the first one, affectivity is more preserved and may manifest as excessive fantasy. In this case, the proximity with 'rich autism' is clear and

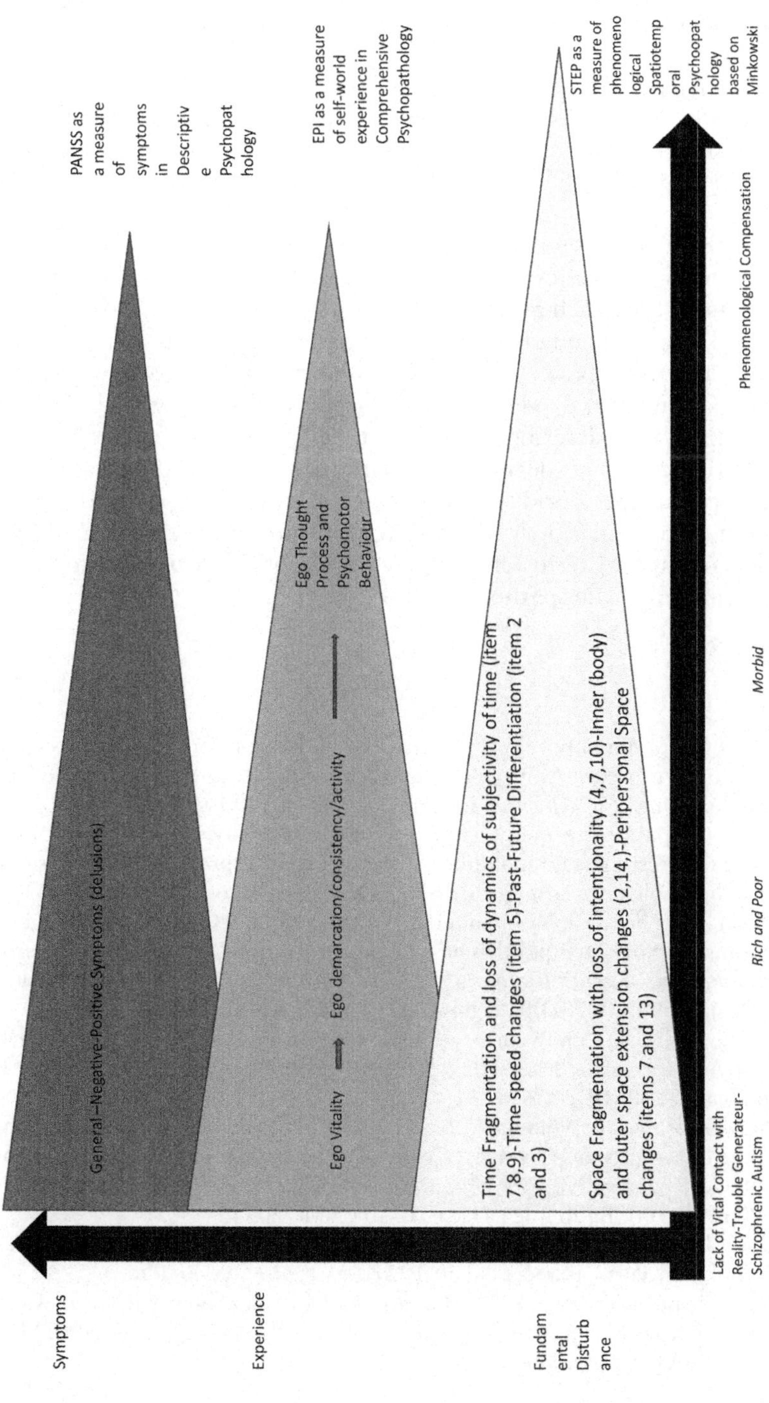

Figure 9.3 Three Layer model about Spatiotemporal Psychopathology on Delusions.

one may assume that the healthy parts of personality are more independent from the fragmented parts;
2. the second type is related to a supra-logical and intellectual attitude. This can be more directly related to morbid rationalism, and, in Minkowski's perspective, it is much more directly influenced by the *trouble générateur*.

In sum, we here conceive delusions and other positive symptoms as secondary or tertiary consequences of an abnormal time-space experience of the world and the own self as part of that world. They are phenomenological and psychological (and ultimately neuronal) compensatory strategies of overcoming the most basic loss of vital contact with reality, that is, the disrupted spatiotemporal relation or connection with the world. That is manifest in the above-described abnormal time-space experience, which, in turn, leads the subject to develop compensatory strategies to regain their vital contact with the world – this is manifest in positive symptoms like delusions and hallucinations. These symptoms are thus explained in primarily spatiotemporal terms entailing what recently has been introduced as Spatiotemporal Psychopathology [1–4].

References

1 Northoff G. Spatiotemporal psychopathology I: No rest for the brain's resting state activity in depression? Spatiotemporal psychopathology of depressive symptoms. *Journal of Affective Disorders* 2016 Jan; 190:854–866.
2 Northoff G. Spatiotemporal psychopathology II: How does a psychopathology of the brain's resting state look like? Spatiotemporal approach and the history of psychopathology. *Journal of Affective Disorders* 2016 Jan; 190:867–879.
3 Northoff G. The brain's spontaneous activity and its psychopathological symptoms – "Spatiotemporal binding and integration". *Progress in Neuro-Psychopharmacology & Biological Psychiatry* 2018 Jan 3;80(Pt B):81–90. doi: 10.1016/j.pnpbp.2017.03.019. Epub 2017 Mar 28. PMID: 28363766.
4 Hirjak D, Wolf RC, Landwehrmeyer GB, Northoff G. Catatonia: looking back and moving forward. *Brain* 2022 Sep 14;145(9):2939–2942. doi: 10.1093/brain/awac196. PMID: 35639851.
5 Arantes-Gonçalves F, Wolman A, Bastos-Leite AJ, Northoff G. Scale for space and time experience in psychosis: Converging phenomenological and psychopathological perspectives. *Psychopathology* 2022;55(3–4):132–142. doi: 10.1159/000519500. Epub 2021 Dec 6. PMID: 34872083.
6 Minkowski E. *La Schizophrénie. Psychopathologie des schizoides et des Schizophrénes*. Paris, France: Payot; 1927.
7 Urfer A. Phenomenology and Psychopathology of Schizophrenia: the views of Eugene Minkowski. *Philosophy, Psychiatry, and Psychology* 2001;8(4):279–289. 10.1353/ppp.2002.0029

8 Abe Y, Raballo A. Minkowski revisited: glancing at the clinical core schizophrenic vulnerability. *Innovations in Clinical Neuroscience* 2013;10(3):10–11.
9 Van Duppen Z. The meaning and relevance of Minkowski's 'loss of vital contact with reality'. *Philosophy, Psychiatry, and Psychology* 2017;24(4):385–397. https://doi.org/10.1353/ppp.2017.0057
10 Minkowski E. Lived Time. In *Phenomenological and Psychopathological Studies* (transl by N Metzel). Evanston, IL: Northwestern University Press, 1970.
11 Kimura B. The Phenomenology of the between: On the Problem of the Basic Disturbance of Schizophrenia. In AJJ De Koning and FA Jenner (eds), *Phenomenology and Psychiatry*. New York: Grune and Sratton. 1982; pp. 173–185.
12 Parnas J, Zandersen M. Can schizophrenia be predicted on the basis of a symptom? A psychopathological appraisal of early detection research in schizophrenia. *Encephale* 2018 Dec;44(6S):S21–S23. doi: 10.1016/S0013-7006(19)30074-0. PMID: 30935482.
13 Zandersen M, Parnas J. Exploring schizophrenia spectrum psychopathology in borderline personality disorder. *European Archives of Psychiatry and Clinical Neuroscience* 2020 Dec;270(8):969–978. doi: 10.1007/s00406-019-01039-4. Epub 2019 Jul 9. PMID: 31289925; PMCID: PMC7599140.
14 Klar P, Northoff G. When the world breaks down: A 3-stage existential model of nihilism in schizophrenia. *Psychopathology* 2021;54(4):169–192. doi: 10.1159/000516814. Epub 2021 Jul 1. PMID: 34198308; PMCID: PMC8619772.
15 Parnas J, Henriksen MG. Disordered self in the schizophrenia spectrum: a clinical and research perspective. *Harvard Review of Psychiatry* 2014 Sep-Oct;22(5):251–265. doi: 10.1097/HRP.0000000000000040. PMID: 25126763; PMCID: PMC4219858.
16 Northoff G, Smith D. The subjectivity of self and its ontology: From the world–brain relation to the point of view in the world. *Theory & Psychology* 2022. https://doi.org/10.1177/09593543221080120
17 Fuchs T, Van Duppen Z. Time and events: On the phenomenology of temporal experience in schizophrenia (Ancillary Article to EAWE Domain 2). *Psychopathology* 2017;50(1):68–74. doi: 10.1159/000452768. Epub 2017 Jan 7. PMID: 28064283.
18 Minkowski E. Findings in a case of schizophrenic depression. 1923. (transl by Barbara Bliss). In Rollo May (ed), *Existence: A New Dimension in Psychiatry and Psychology*. New York, NY: Basic Books, 1958; pp. 127–138.
19 Stanghellini G, Fernandez AV, Ballerini M, Blasi S, Belfiore E, Cutting J, Mancini M. Abnormal space experiences in persons with schizophrenia: An empirical qualitative study. *Schizophrenia Bulletin* 2020 Apr 10;46(3):530–539. doi: 10.1093/schbul/sbz107. PMID: 31784743; PMCID: PMC7147594.
20 Thönes S, Stocker K. A standard conceptual framework for the study of subjective time. *Consciousness and Cognition* 2019 May;71:114–122. doi: 10.1016/j.concog.2019.04.004. Epub 2019 Apr 17. PMID: 31004875.
21 Stanghellini G, Ballerini M, Presenza S, Mancini M, Raballo A, Blasi S, Cutting J. Psychopathology of lived time: Abnormal time experience in persons with schizophrenia. *Schizophrenia Bulletin* 2016 Jan;42(1):45–55. doi: 10.1093/schbul/sbv052. Epub 2015 May 4. PMID: 25943123; PMCID: PMC4681541.

22 Palumbo D, Stanghellini G, Mucci A, Ballerini M, Giordano GM, Lysaker PH, Galderisi S. Autism rating scale: A new tool for characterizing the schizophrenia phenotype. *Frontiers in Psychiatry* 2021 Jan 26;12:622359. doi: 10.3389/fpsyt.2021.622359. PMID: 33574776; PMCID: PMC7870791.
23 Fuchs, T. Temporality and psychopathology. *Phenomenology and the Cognitive Sciences* 2013 12;75–104. doi: 10.1007/s11097-010-9189-4

10 Defining Delusion in the DSM-5

Jorge Gonçalves

Introduction

In the current psychiatric literature, "delusion" is defined as a symptom that appears in several syndromes. Psychiatry is a science that emerged in a certain historical period (see Foucault et al. 2006), and its findings and tenets reflect specific social and ontological values (Sadler, 2013). We should thus regard the knowledge gleaned by this science not as timeless and definitive but as relative to a certain social and scientific context.

Philosophy and psychiatry each take a different approach to delusions, although they can help each other. As a branch of medicine, psychiatry seeks above all to distinguish between the *normal* and the *pathological* and to establish therapies that help subjects to alleviate their psychological suffering. Philosophy studies delusion as a mental state in a more neutral way, regardless of whether the delusion has pathological consequences or not. However, here I will be mainly concerned with clinical delusions, that is, those that have been brought to the attention of psychiatrists and clinical psychologists. Even in this context, however, philosophy, which is less bound to immediate practical application, can be useful for psychiatry, helping it to develop greater conceptual rigor.

The definitions provided in psychiatry manuals allow for the identification of problematic behavior in those who seek professional help for their mental problems. The definition of "delusion", according to the most influential manual—the DSM-5—is as follows:

> A false belief based on incorrect inference about external reality that is firmly held despite what almost everyone else believes and despite what constitutes incontrovertible and obvious proof or evidence to the contrary. The belief is not ordinarily accepted by other members of the

DOI: 10.4324/9781003288992-14

> person's culture or subculture (i.e., it is not an article of religious faith). When a false belief involves a value judgment, it is regarded as a delusion only when the judgment is so extreme as to defy credibility.
>
> (American Psychiatric Association, 2013: 819)

From the third edition onwards, the DSM has aimed to describe symptoms in an objective and atheoretical way. The two previous editions were strongly influenced by a psychoanalytic model that relativized both the importance and the process of diagnosis. It was found that the diagnosis could vary greatly depending on the clinician. To overcome this, an attempt was made to create an instrument that would gather broad consensus and that did not rely on previous explanatory guidance. In principle, the DSM provides objective data that is prior to and independent of any particular neurocognitive, psychodynamic or any other model. This objective is an ideal, however, and in reality an implicit position is always taken. The above definition of delusion contains several implicit assumptions, which have since been questioned. José E. Porcher (cf. Porcher, 2016) has summarized these questions as follows: Are delusions beliefs, or are they another state of mind/propositional attitude? Must delusions be false? Must they be based on inference? Do delusions necessarily have to be about external reality? Need they be firmly sustained? Do all delusions occur in the face of incontrovertible and obvious proof or evidence to the contrary? Must they contradict what almost everyone else believes? Does the attribution of delusion have to take into consideration the person's culture or subculture?

Here, we will focus on the first claim: that *delusion is a false belief*. The question that arises is whether we can attribute to delusional states the status of belief, which may lead to the question of the *nature of belief*. Although they are related, however, the former question is different from the latter.

First, however, we should note that in the definition of delusion what is at stake is not what reality itself is but the relationship between the individual's beliefs and the beliefs of his community. The beliefs held by the individual suffering from delusion(s) are obviously false in the eyes of society. In this way, social or communal beliefs are excluded from being delusions—for example shared religious beliefs that, although in conflict with science, are accepted by vast members of society.

Why have psychiatrists traditionally classified delusions as beliefs? One of the reasons could be that this is what gives them their pathological character. Commonly, delusions are first noticed by those closest to the subject: family, friends, and colleagues. What is shocking to people is that the subject seems to believe "obviously absurd" things with great conviction. If the subject were to accept that his claims were the product of his imagination, they would not be considered pathological delusions. It is the fact that the subject is convinced of what he says that makes him "crazy" in the eyes of others. It seems, therefore, that when the subject is deluded, he accepts his claims as true.

Several critiques have been voiced against the quite common-sense idea that delusion is a belief. According to some philosophers of mind (see Graham, 2020 and Bortolotti, 2010), in order to ascribe belief status to a mental state, certain requirements must be fulfilled. If the delusion does not meet these requirements, it should be considered not a belief but another type of mental state. In Anglo-American philosophy of mind, belief has been defined as a propositional attitude, that is, an attitude we have towards an explicit or implicit proposition. This attitude of "belief" consists in intending that the proposition is true, that is, that it corresponds to the situation in the world.

If I believe in the proposition "Russian troops have entered Ukraine", I think this is what is happening in the world. If I care about the truth of that belief, I will try to make sure it is true. For example, I will try to make sure that the source of the information is reliable. Some philosophers then developed the theory that there is an intimate relationship between belief and rationality. If a belief is really a belief, then it must not contradict the empirical data and the subject's other beliefs. If a contradiction can be shown, then the subject must abandon the belief on pain of irrationality. I once thought that a certain philosopher had already passed away of old age. Someone showed me proof that this philosopher was alive, and so I abandoned my belief, even though it took me a while to publicly acknowledge my mistake.

Lisa Bortolotti (2010) distinguishes three types of rationality associated with beliefs: *procedural rationality* (the integration of beliefs and other propositional attitudes held by the subject); *epistemic rationality* (the belief must be in harmony with the available evidence); and *agentive rationality* (beliefs must justify the subject's actions). At least some delusions are found to violate these rational norms. The delusion often does not have the consequences it would have if the subject really believed it. This has led researchers to claim that delusional states cannot be equated with the propositional attitude of "belief". Several alternatives have been proposed: some think that delusions have no meaning and are mere utterances of meaningless words. Others maintain that the question should be referred to neuroscience rather than the philosophy of mind. Others argue that delusions are experiences, not beliefs. Still others have proposed different types of mental states that are not recognized in folk psychology.

Bortolotti and Miyazono (leading specialists in the field) acknowledge the variety of theoretical accounts of delusion:

> Although some argue that delusions are empty utterances with no meaning (Berrios), most anti-doxasticists defend the view that delusions are mental states of a non-doxastic or a non-exclusively-doxastic nature: acts of imagination (Currie and Ravenscroft; Currie and Jureidini), perceptual inferences (Hohwy and Rajan), states in-between beliefs and non-beliefs (Schwitzgebel; Tumulty), states in-between beliefs and desires or in-between beliefs and imaginings (Egan), attitudes towards mental states (Stephens and Graham), acceptances (Frankish) or thoughts expressing the content of default processes (Gerrans).
>
> (Bortolotti and Miyazono, 2015)

In this chapter, I approach delusional states (as described in both the DSM-5 and elsewhere) from an anti-rationalist standpoint, defending a broad notion of "belief" that includes irrational episodes.

Defense of the Doxastic Position

One way of arguing that delusions are beliefs is to point out that delusions do not always violate the norms of rationality. For example, there are cases of subjects who argue in defense of their delusions and others who act according to their delusions. There are also known cases of subjects who change their delusions in light of empirical evidence or rational arguments. Can one then say that delusions are like other beliefs, only slightly disturbed by motivational or other factors? One could accept this solution without questioning the rationality of belief, since delusion does not violate rationality on this view. In this sense, this solution would be compatible with the theory that relates rationality to belief. It is not a good solution, however, because many delusions do not in fact respect these rational norms. If we accept that responsiveness to such norms is a necessary condition for belief, then delusions cannot be beliefs. At the very least, most known delusions would remain unexplained.

Another, more convincing argument in favor of the view that delusions are beliefs involves questioning whether beliefs are as rational as philosophers of mind claim. What we in common parlance designate as 'belief states' do not always fulfill the rules of rationality set out above. A man who piously believes in the words of the Gospel while attending Mass can have sinful thoughts as soon as he enters the atrium. Many people believe in so-called superstitions even though they follow a scientific way of thinking in other situations. Others hold empirically groundless prejudices against certain peoples and social groups. It can easily be seen that these beliefs violate the types of rationality defined by Bortolotti and mentioned above. In this case, the difference between beliefs and delusions would seem to be one of degree rather than one of kind. Indeed, this approach envisages a continuum with rational, scientific beliefs at one extreme, delusions at the other, and hypocrisy, superstition, and prejudice somewhere in the middle. This model also has therapeutic consequences, thus making delusions accessible to cognitive behavioral therapy and psychodynamics.

One objection to this view is that delusion becomes trivialized, treated as an extravagant belief. In response, one might again point out that religious beliefs are sometimes also very extravagant from a scientific worldview. In Catholicism, it is believed that Jesus died and rose again and that pieces of bread are transformed into his body every Sunday. Millions of people hold this belief, and from a naturalistic point of view it is very strange, but still a belief. Likewise, a delusion that is held as a personal, unshared, even bizarre conviction does not cease to be a belief for that reason. The notion of "bizarreness" is relative to sociocultural contexts.

Delusions as Experiences

Phenomenologists have mainly concerned themselves with psychotic delusions, but their conclusions can perhaps be extended to other types of delusions. Psychotic delusions sometimes resemble metaphysical or political explanatory systems (Bentall, 2018) in the sense that they aim to explain the totality of reality. Authors who defend such a view are concerned not so much with explaining the formation of delusions as with exploring how they manifest themselves as data of consciousness. Phenomenology, a philosophical method developed by Husserl, Heidegger, Sartre, and others, aims to describe things as they appear to the subject, prior to the adoption of any one explanatory theory. Applied to psychiatry, this method is based on empathy, or immediate knowledge of the mental states of the other (see Gonçalves, 2019).

Shaun Gallagher, for example, bases his approach to delusions on Alfred Schutz's model, according to which, in addition to everyday states of consciousness, consciousness can enter other states: religion, fiction, dream (Gallagher, 2015, 2009). These states are described as "realities" rather than unreal deviations. They are incommensurable, they do not communicate with each other, and the passage from one to the other takes place by leaps. When consciousness finds itself in an alternate reality, it is not just an inner change; it is the whole of reality that is transformed. For example, in the dream state we enter "another world" which is not governed by the laws of our everyday world. When we move from the dream to everyday reality, we make a "leap" to a new reality. Delusion is also a real experience that does not just happen in the subject's mind, since, for him, all of reality is transformed. Objects in the world acquire new affordances in a delusional state. Delusion is an alternative reality, not a mere false belief. The subject lives partly in the world of delusion and partly in the world of everyday consciousness. In this way, it is possible to understand the contradictions in which the subject seems to enter, with the passage from reality-as-delusion to the reality of common sense.

Another influential phenomenologist who has studied delusion, Louis Sass (cf. Sass, 1995), provides a detailed description of the schizophrenic's world experience, based on the text "Memories of My Nervous Illness" by Daniel Paul Schreber, the most famous case of psychotic delusion to date (and initially studied by Freud).[1] Schreber elaborated a complex cosmogony accompanied by visual and auditory hallucinations. From this case, Sass generalizes to delusions in general. He does not claim that his perspective explains all delusions, but it can be helpful for understanding a good many of them. His interpretation differs from mainstream psychoanalysis in several respects. For the purposes of this article, it is important to point out that he thinks that delusion should not be defined in terms of a failure to pass the so-called reality test. At least some psychotics do not fail to recognize common social reality. This is evident in the so-called double bookkeeping phenomenon identified by Bleuler (1950), an example of which is the psychiatric patient who accuses the hospital of poisoning his food but who continues to eat it. On Sass's reading, the patient does not fail the reality test. He knows the food is not poisoned. Sometimes he even gives off the impression of being ironic, as if to say, "I'm not being serious, don't you know that?"

Phenomenologists, then, argue that delusion should be defined not in contrast to social reality but as an experience in its own right. The delusional subject knows common social reality and knows how to move within it; at the same time, however, he cannot avoid the delusional experience that is imposed on his conscience. The delusion is therefore not a belief; it is an experience, and as an experience it cannot be true or false. If a person takes a psychedelic drug and has a certain mental experience, we cannot say that this experience is true or false – only whether it exists or not.

However, the idea that delusion is an experience is not incompatible with its also being a belief. A belief can be generated from an experience, regardless of the origin and formation of that experience. The origin and formation of the experience may be motivational or neurological, but here we are only interested in highlighting that the experience may be the basis of belief. On Freud's interpretation (Freud, 2014/1911), it was the experience of repressed homosexuality that gave rise to Schreber's delusion. Others may argue that it was due to neurological alterations. In any case, internal experiences spurred Schreber's delusional state.

If a person takes LSD and then describes his experience—say, seeing people with frogs' heads—as very interesting, we would not view him as "crazy". However, if he says that he has begun to realize that people actually have frogs' heads, that they are likely aliens, and so on, he will begin to be regarded with suspicion. Where does the difference lie? In the first case, the person had an experience that did not produce belief, while in the second the experience modified his beliefs. Therefore, it is the belief aspect that determines the pathological character of the delusion. In this sense, viewing delusions as experiences does not preclude also viewing them as beliefs.

Gallagher seems to assume that the difference between belief and experience lies in the degree of control (see Gallagher, 2009, p. 257). An experience involves the individual's entire being, being irrefutable as an experience. Belief is something that the subject can change according to empirical evidence and arguments. However, the fact that belief imposes itself and resists change does not entail that it is not belief. One can see this in certain religious and political beliefs. Arguments against the existence of God have little effect on what we call "faith", that is, belief against the available data. The religious believer sees absence of evidence as proof of the purity of his faith. There would be no merit in believing in God if He manifested himself in an evident way.

Are Beliefs Reducible to Neuronal States?

Some authors argue that the discussion about whether delusions are beliefs is not very interesting insofar as "belief" is a term from popular psychology and, when a neurological explanation is reached, we can dispense with popular psychology concepts. We can continue to use these concepts in our daily lives, but we should not consider them for the purposes of scientific explanation. I think that here one must distinguish between reflection on ultimate reality, that is, metaphysics, and useful psychological explanation.

From a metaphysical point of view, one can admit that the ultimate level of reality is matter/energy. There is, however, still the so-called hard problem of consciousness, which I will not discuss here, and which raises questions about the reduction of mind to matter/energy (Chalmers, 1995). From a point of view that is useful to psychology and psychiatry, however, there are several levels of description of human behavior, which one can divide into the personal and the sub-personal. Neuroscience has made great advances at the sub-personal level, which sustains the personal sphere. In acknowledging these advances, however, we should not forget that the description of human behavior begins at the level of consciousness, language, and social relations. A mental disorder only makes sense as a behavioral (including linguistic behavior) deviation from what is expected in each society. Usually, delusions are detected at the linguistic level. It is the speech of the subject who, in the social environment in which he is inserted, violates the expected rules of rationality that helps us to diagnose delusions. Take, for example, the woman who says, "This man is not my husband; he is an imposter" (Capgras delusion). This sentence, which expresses a belief, is well constructed from a syntactic point of view. It has a problem, however: it does not correspond to the empirical reality that everyone observes. This is where the process of attributing delusion begins: with a false belief that resists all contrary arguments. This attribution of belief considers the social reality in which the subject is inserted.

Only then does the process of trying to explain the delusion begin. In the example, the first explanations were motivational, within a psychodynamic model. However, it was found that a neurocognitive model is more plausible (McKay, Langdon, and Coltheart, 2007), although the motivational model may still have importance, alongside mixed models (*idem*). Not all delusions necessarily have neurological alterations (*idem*), but if we consider only those that do, this does not mean that the level of belief is reduced or eliminated.

Neurology serves to explain what happens in human reality, which is also a social reality, where interpersonal relationships are present. In either situation, the level of consciousness and intentionality is necessary for an understanding of human behavior that is useful to psychiatry and clinical psychology. Our knowledge is not, and likely will never be, at a level where neurology alone is able to draw conclusions about the mental state of the subject, especially since the subject's mental state and behavior depend on social factors that cannot be reduced to neurology. For example, studies show that migrants are more prone to psychotic disorders than other people. Although neurology can also play a role here, the causes stem more from a social situation that can modify neural circuits in the brains of those subject to delusions.

One of the authors who criticizes the doxastic position is Philip Gerrans. He writes:

> Thus, a good theoretical definition is one that ensures that investigators at all levels of a mechanism's function are talking about the same thing. It follows that such definitions are provisional and revisable. The definitions of delusion in the DSM-IV and V made this integrative type of explanation impossible precisely because they deal in folk psychological notions (incorrect inference) that seem to apply exclusively at the personal level. … It is not clear that DSM definitions are intended as theoretical definitions in my required sense rather than a clinical heuristic, or regimentation of everyday intuitions that inevitably build in

> normative notion[s] of rationality. In the absence of any alternative, however, theorists often use the clinical definition as a basis for theoretical definition.
>
> (Gerrans, 2014, p. 36)

Gerrans's model is *integrative*, holding that the nervous system has several levels of control over information, each level supervising the previous one. The personal level of consciousness, intentionality and language is not eliminated from the system. However, he argues that one cannot always preserve the terms of folk psychology at the scientific level, because these terms do not integrate well with the explanation of the other, sub-personal levels. In this sense, he does not define delusion as "false belief". His definition of delusion states that "[d]elusions arise when default cognitive processing, unsupervised by decontextualized processing, is monopolized by hypersalient information" (Gerrans, 2014, p. 38).

Default cognitive processing is the processing of information by the Default Mode Network (DMN), a brain structure that is used to simulate and solve problems without action, only in the mind, in so-called mental time travel. When it is not solving problems, the DMN keeps working, producing autobiographical fragments and personal narratives, that is, a purely subjective treatment of information. The DMN is in turn supervised by another neural system, the dorsolateral prefrontal cortex (DLPFC), which treats the information in a decontextualized way. This information is used publicly and no longer merely subjectively. That is to say, we are almost always producing subjective and autobiographical narrative fragments about the inputs that come to us from perception and sensory data. If we stick to this information, we dive into subjective states that can be dreams or delusions, with differences between them. We then need to submit the information elaborated by the DMN to the decontextualization process carried out by the dorsolateral prefrontal cortex. The decontextualization of information underlies activities such as logical reasoning, consulting maps, and so on. We stop seeing from a subjective point of view and tend to situate ourselves within a "view from nowhere" (to use Thomas Nagel's terminology). On Gerrans's model, these possibilities for processing information reside in brain structures, and damage to these structures may produce abnormal situations. By *salience* (in the above definition) Gerrans means the allocation of resources in adaptively important information. At the personal level, one speaks of attention, concentration, and the like, and there are neurological equivalents at the sub-personal level. As can be seen from the definition, in delusion an abnormal process is at work.

How is delusion explained on this model? DMN and DLPFC are *anti-correlated*: when one is very active, the other is less active. When the DMN produces subjective information not controlled by the DLPFC, we say that the subject is out of reality. There is a normal process in life where this happens, that is, when we are dreaming. Here, there is a break with the rest of psychic reality, and autobiographical narrative fragments parade freely, overlapping with one another without any attempt to apply themselves to the solution of a problem. In delusion there is involvement with the rest of psychic reality, and delusions lack the sharp disconnection from social reality that we find in dreams. In schizophrenic delusions, the DMN is hyperactive, and the DLPFC cannot decontextualize the information. In delusions such as Capgras, which are monothematic, the DMN is not hyperactive, but due to damage to the DLPFC, the production of subjective fragments is not decontextualized and statements become purely subjective, without concern for what others say. The subject does not realize that the notion "my husband is an imposter" is just a subjective impression. She does not confront this subjective impression with decontextualized knowledge, the cause of which is an internal injury.

Gerrans distinguishes his model from those that view delusions as resulting from a failure in the belief evaluation mechanism (Coltheart, Langdon, & McKay, 2011; Coltheart, Menzies, & Sutton, 2010). According to these authors, delusion is a belief generated in response to a bizarre experience caused by certain brain injuries. This is rational, but it is no longer rational when compared to other evidence: what others say, empirical evidence, and so on. A woman recognizes her husband's face, but she does not feel the familiarity she used to feel. To explain this phenomenon, she claims that he is an imposter, which seems to be rational. However, when confronted with all the other evidence, she stubbornly remains committed to her belief, which can be explained by damage to a part of the brain used for evaluating beliefs. According to Coltheart, Menzies, and Sutton (2010), this is likely a lateral region of the right frontal cortex.

However, Gerrans argues that the narrative productions of the DMN should not be called "beliefs" but rather "imaginations". Belief for him implies procedural rationality (see above), which would then be the measure of madness. Yet if one follows Bortolotti's idea (cf. Bortolotti & Gunn 2016) that beliefs need not necessarily be rational, can one accept that Gerrans's model is compatible with the doxastic model? And what would be the interest of establishing this compatibility? The interest would be that in psychiatry and clinical psychology the concept of mental illness/disorder is not disconnected from social common sense. There is interest in having a description that is useable by the public or in a judicial context, for example. I will say more about this later. Gerrans's definition is scientific, and I think it is only incompatible with the doxastic model if we think that the idealized version of rational belief is the only true one. Yet if we attribute the status of belief to non-coherent and irrational states, we can accept that the integrative model does not eliminate the doxastic model. The choice of one or another mode of description will have to do with the objectives of that description in social contexts. *Gerrans's integrative model requires that descriptions at the personal level be integrable with those at the neuronal level.* However, in many social practices, we do not need to descend to these levels to communicate. On the other hand, given the subtlety of human psychology, we may wonder whether the personal level and the neuronal level will ever be integrable without loss of information.

Are Delusions Beliefs, or Are They Acceptances?

The attribution of belief to delusional people originates not in scientific theory but in folk psychology, understood as the spontaneous psychology that everyone uses, even if they have never read anything about scientific psychology. However, we can ask whether the concept of "belief" is perhaps like the concept of "consciousness", which covers different types of mental states, as suggested by Ned Block (Block, 2002).

Some authors have proposed a revision of the relevant concepts, making the analysis more refined. They argue that popular psychology emerged in the context of neurotypical people and that in the case of mental disturbances, other terms are necessary, such as acts of imagination, perceptual inferences, states in-between belief and non-belief, states in-between belief and desire or in-between belief and imaginings, attitudes towards mental states, acceptances or thoughts that express the content of default processes, and the like.

Richard Dub (Dub, 2017) argues that doxastic arguments against the revised concepts mentioned above are valid because criticisms of the doxastic model have been purely conceptual rather than explanatory. He writes: "I call these 'conceptual' arguments because the first premise is often justified through a priori conceptual analysis: analysis of BELIEF tells us something about the necessary features of belief" (Dub, 2013, p. 33). Dub's main thesis is that delusions are really *acceptances*, generated by pathologically powerful cognitive feelings.

The doxastic model would continue to have difficulties explaining, above all, the situations Dub designates as *circumscription* and *double bookkeeping*. As he puts it: "The odd features of delusions are explained in want of a theory. My goal is to provide a model that can give explanations and provide understanding where current doxasticist models cannot" (Dub, 2017, p. 35).

The first phenomenon—circumscription—refers to the relative inertness of delusions in affecting cognition and behavior. Double bookkeeping, on the other hand, also known as "double registration", refers to a phenomenon first identified by the early Eugen Bleuler (1950) and written about at length by Louis Sass (1995). Delusional subjects appear to keep two "books" or "registries" of representations in their heads—one of "the real world" and one of "the delusional world"—and they are able to keep these books reasonably well partitioned. Surprisingly, delusional individuals often speak as if they were aware that they are operating on the basis of two different sets of representations: they speak of their "delusional reality" and can identify which of their mental states are delusional.

Dub proposes a model for explaining such situations. His model builds on Frankish's (Frankish, 2004, 2009, 2011), although there are differences between them. According to this model, delusions are acceptances. What are acceptances? For Frankish (see Bauman, 2011), the term came from philosophers of science. Van Fraasen (see *idem*) maintains that a scientist can defend as true a theory about which there may be doubt. Take, for example, the social scientist who maintains that Marxism is true while knowing full well that there are many questions about it. He will thus be able to analyze social facts on the basis of Marxist assumptions. Dub says it is unrealistic to give a definition of acceptance, but he aims to make the notion clearer through several examples. In a first approximation, acceptance is like an assumption or presupposition, but it remains in the mind and is incorporated into an individual's thinking, becoming a premise of his reasoning. An example of this (not Dub's own) is a person who wants to enter politics but is undecided about which party to choose. Noting that he has a better chance of reaching the top in a certain party, he decides to adhere to the ideas of that party – ideas in which he does not fully believe but which he defends vehemently in debates, rallies, official communiqués, and so on. Over the years, he gradually forgets that his initial adherence to the party's ideas was but a means to an end, and at some point, although he continues to have many doubts about the correctness of these ideas, he fully accepts them. If given to introspection, he would say that deep down he never believed in the party's core ideas but that for the sake of his career, he accepted its ideology. If not given to introspection, he would say: "Of course I always believed them". According to Dub, what this individual has is an acceptance and not a belief. However, it would be belief if his belief system validated this acceptance (which, hypothetically, it does not).

To be able to affirm that delusions are acceptances, however, Dub adds a modification to the usual theories on the subject. Theorists usually consider acceptances to be voluntary and conscious, not unconscious and involuntary, like beliefs. Dub bases his model on dual theories, according to which there are two types of information processing: "type 1" processes are typically thought to be fast, parallel, unconscious, automatic, and associative; "type 2" processes are evolutionarily younger and are performed by systems that are uniquely human; these processes are slow, conscious, serial, rule-governed, and domain-general. Acceptances are processed by type 2 and beliefs by type 1 processes.

Delusions are involuntary, however, and thus Dub must admit that although acceptances are typically voluntary, they are not always so. As he claims:

> Most standing states of acceptance might be formed through voluntary action, but some cases – pathological cases of acceptance such as delusion would be particularly good candidates – might well involve involuntary acceptance fixation. An arm movement can be either volitional or the result of a spasm; a mental movement can similarly be either volitional or not.
>
> (Dub, 2017, p. 46)

Delusions are pathological acceptances caused by the so-called cognitive feelings that the author describes. In short, they are feelings through which we become aware of our epistemic situation. These feelings generate acceptances, not beliefs. If I see a person and feel that he is familiar, I accept that he is a familiar person, and I treat him as such. Such cognitive feelings include: a feeling of understanding, a feeling of safety, a feeling of importance, and a feeling of familiarity. When they result from brain lesions, these feelings can be pathological and generate delusions, with different elaborations.

Which of the two descriptions of delusion—*belief* or *acceptance*—should we adopt? We may try to determine which is more accurate, that is, which best fits reality, or we may think that both descriptions are acceptable and that the choice depends on pragmatic considerations. In this second case, one may take a clinical point of view according to which it is better to use the term "belief", as a word that is commonly used and understood in everyday life. Practitioners, patients, and their families will intuitively understand the concept of "false belief". This intuition comes from the fact that we all know deep down that we have irrational beliefs and that delusion is just a more extreme case of such beliefs.

As for Dub's model, I think he remains stuck in the idealized model of philosophy of mind, according to which beliefs must be rational if they are to be beliefs. Cases of circumscription and double bookkeeping can be explained as irrational beliefs. In everyday life, we often seek to rationalize the irrational. If we accept the psychoanalytic model and hold that there are motives that the subject cannot access via introspection, we can explain the irrationality of certain beliefs. However, even if we reject the psychoanalytic model, we can accept commonsense concepts such as "laziness", "hypocrisy", and so on as forms of explanation.

I see no reason to think that a delusional individual does not believe the contents of his delusion. To the extent that he has other beliefs that collide with it, he seems to demonstrate that he does not have the unity and coherence that he imagines himself to have. Dub states that the irrational beliefs of neurotypicals are not really beliefs but acceptances. He continues: "Bortolotti is correct that neurotypical subjects have mental states that are similar to delusions, but this does not mean that delusions are beliefs. It could also mean that atypical 'beliefs' in neurotypical subjects turn out not to be beliefs" (Dub, 2017, p. 35).

It seems to me, therefore, that Dub is committed to the theory that beliefs are necessarily rational. Dub thus asserts that although folk psychology views beliefs as mental states that approach delusions, we are not bound to accept this explanation. As we have seen, popular psychology was not designed to give scientific explanations, and in the case of delusion one must have a finer analysis of belief. Hence, Dub resorted to the concept of acceptances. However, his critique is based on the theory that there is a necessary link between beliefs and rationality. If one accepts that beliefs can be irrational, is it necessary to complicate the doxastic model? I think that the departure from popular psychology is only justified when it proves to be insufficient, which is not the case here.

Conclusion

If one accepts this doxastic model, according to which beliefs can be irrational, one must admit that our beliefs do not have the rationality we imagine they do. The Portuguese poet Fernando Pessoa even made this a positive principle:

> If there is a strange and inexplicable fact, it is that a creature of intelligence and sensitivity always remains seated on the same opinion, always consistent with itself. The continuous transformation of everything also takes place in the body, and consequently takes place in the brain. How then, if not through illness, to fall and relapse into the abnormality of wanting to think the same thing today as was thought yesterday, when not only is today's brain no longer yesterday's, but today is not yesterday?
>
> (Pessoa, 1915)

Pessoa may be exaggerating slightly here, but it is nonetheless true that our beliefs often lack internal coherence and do not cease to be beliefs because of that. A possible explanation for why beliefs do not always follow the patterns of rationality described above relates to the fact that beliefs are linked to motives, emotions, and experiences. A person who generally thinks that it's better to deal with issues right away, for instance, may sometimes put things off because they are related to painful emotions he doesn't want to face. Belief in this case has nothing to do with proper behavior. Racist beliefs are another example of attitudes that are held without rational verification and that would in fact fail to align with reason were they examined.

In neurotypical people, the contradictions among their beliefs are not very serious, and they try to correct them (as in so-called cognitive dissonance) (Bortolotti, 2010). Faced with two dissonant beliefs, the subject can create a conceptualization that reconciles them. One experiment (Festinger, Riecken, and Schachter, 1956) studied members of a religious sect who believed that the world would end on a certain day. When that day came and the world did not end, they tried to come up with an alternative explanation. There are also contradictions that people are not aware of and that are not very important in practical life.

Why, then, does the subject shift from moderate contradictions to true absurdities and delusion? Here arise theories concerning the formation of delusions: motivational, neurocognitive, and others, which I will not address in this article. The doxastic model holds that delusions can be described as beliefs but does not explain why such irrational beliefs arise in the subject. Bortolotti hypothesizes that these are extreme cases of irrationality with, as we have seen, continuity between normal beliefs and delusions. In my view, we do not currently need a theory about the formation of delusions that explains everything, at least at this stage of knowledge of the human mind. The problem with psychoanalysis, rational cognitive therapy, and neuroscience is sometimes that they want to explain all delusions, when delusions may have different causes. Where one delusion may be caused by a subject's not wanting to accept his own homosexual tendencies, another may have its origin in an injury to the brain. In the current state of our knowledge of delusions, these different theories should be seen as hypotheses to be developed. From a clinical point of view, criticism has arisen concerning the economic interests at stake in this area (e.g., the interests of pharmaceutical companies, psychology departments, and the like), which risk undermining the disinterested study of the phenomenon of delusion.

Note

1 According to Bleuler, Schreber was a schizophrenic; according to Freud, he was suffering from paranoia.

References

American Psychiatric Association (2013). DSM-5, p. 819.

Baumann, P. (2011). Empiricism, stances, and the problem of voluntarism. *Synthese* 178, 27–36. https://doi.org/10.1007/s11229-009-9519-7

Bentall, R.P. (2018). Delusions and other beliefs. In Bortolotti, L. (Ed.), *Delusions in Context*. Palgrave Macmillan, Cham.

Bleuler, E. (1950). *Dementia Praecox or the Group of Schizophrenias* (trans. J. Zinkin & N. D. C. Lewis). International University Press, New York (Original work published 1911).

Block, Ned (2002). Some concepts of consciousness. In Chalmers, D. (Ed.), *Philosophy of Mind: Classical and Contemporary Readings*, pp. 206–219.

Bortolotti, L. (2010). *Delusions and Other Irrational Beliefs.* Oxford University Press, Oxford.

Bortolotti, L. & Miyazono, K. (2015). Recent work on the nature and development of delusions philosophy. *Compass* 10(9), 636–645.

Bortolotti, L., & Gunn, R. (2016). Review of the measure of madness: Philosophy of mind, cognitive neuroscience, and delusional thought, by P. GERRANS. *The British Journal for the Philosophy of Science* 67(3), 919–923. http://www.jstor.org/stable/43946100

Chalmers, D.J. (1995). Facing up to the problem of consciousness. *Journal of Consciousness Studies* 2, 200–219.

Coltheart, M., Langdon, R. & McKay, R. Jan (2011). Delusional belief. *Annual Review of Psychology* 62, 271–298.

Coltheart, M., Menzies, P., & Sutton, J. (2010). Abductive inference and delusional belief. *Cognitive Neuropsychiatry* 15, 261–287.

Dub, R. (2013). Dissertation Thesis. New Brunswick, New Jersey. 03-10-2022.

Dub, R. (2017). Delusions, acceptances, and cognitive feelings. *Philosophy and Phenomenological Research* 94, 27–60.

Festinger, Leon, Riecken, Henry W., & Schachter, Stanley (1956). *When Prophecy Fails: A Social and Psychological Study of a Modern Group that Predicted the Destruction of the World.* University of Minnesota Press. ISBN 1-59147-727-1. Reissued 2008 by Pinter & Martin with a foreword by Elliot Aronson, ISBN 978-1-905177-19-6

Foucault, M., Lagrange, J., Ewald, F., Fontana, A., & Davidson, A. I. (Eds.). (2006). *Michel Foucault: Psychiatric Power: Lectures at the Collège de France, 1973–1974.* (G. Burchell, Trans.). Palgrave Macmillan, London.

Frankish, K. (2004). *Mind and Supermind.* Cambridge University Press, Cambridge.

Frankish, K. (2009). Delusions: A two-level framework. In Broome, M. R. & Bortolotti, L. (Eds.), *Psychiatry as Cognitive Neuroscience: Philosophical Perspectives, International Perspectives in Philosophy and Psychiatry.* Oxford University Press, Oxford.

Frankish, K. 2011. Delusions, levels of belief, and nondoxastic acceptances. *Neuroethics.* https://doi.org/10.1007/s12152-011-9123-7

Freud, S. (1911, 1958). *Psycho-Analytic Notes on an Autobiographical Account of a Case of Paranoia (Dementia Paranoides).* In The Standard Edition of the Complete Psychological Works of Sigmund Freud (Trans. James Strachey). Vol. XII (1911–1913). The Hogarth Press and the Institute of Psychoanalysis, London.

Gallagher, S. (2015). Why we are not all novelists. In Bundgaard, P. F. and Stjernfelt, F. (Eds.), *Investigations into the Phenomenology and the Ontology of the Work of Art: What are Artworks and How Do We Experience Them?* SpringerOpen, London, pp. 129–143.

Gallagher, S. (2009). Delusional realities. In Broome, M.R. & Bortolotti, L. (Eds.), *Psychiatry as Cognitive Neuroscience: Philosophical Perspectives*. Oxford University Press, Oxford, pp. 245–266.

Gerrans, P. (2014). *The Measure of Madness: Philosophy of Mind, Cognitive Neuroscience, and Delusional Thought*. MIT Press, Cambridge, MA.

Gonçalves, J. (2019). Intersubjectivity in psychiatry. In *Phenomenological Approaches to Intersubjectivity and Values*. Cambridge Scholars Publishing, Newcastle-upon-Tyne.

Graham, G. (2020). *The Disordered Mind* (3rd ed.). Routledge. Taylor and Francis, London.

McKay, R., Langdon, R. & Coltheart, M. (2007). Models of misbelief: Integrating motivational and deficit theories of delusions. *Consciousness and Cognition* 16(4), 932–941

Pessoa, F. (1915). Crónica da vida que passa. in O Jornal, n° 2. Lisboa: 5-4-191530-09-2022 http://arquivopessoa.net/textos/3413

Porcher, J.P. (2016). The classification, definition, and ontology of delusion. *Revista Latinoamericana de Psicopatologia Fundamental* 19, 167–181.

Sadler, J. Z. (2013). Values in psychiatric diagnosis and classification. In Fulford, K. W. M., Davies, M., Gipps, R. G. T., Graham, G., Sadler, J. Z., Stanghellini, G., & Thornton, T. (Eds.), *The Oxford Handbook of Philosophy and Psychiatry*. Oxford University Press, Oxford, pp. 753–778.

Sass, L. (1995). The paradoxes of delusion. In *Wittgenstein, Schreber, and the Schizophrenic Mind*. Cornell University Press, Ithaca, New York, and London (first published in 1994).

11 Delusions across and beyond Diagnoses

Luigi Grassi and Lisa Bortolotti

Introduction

In this chapter, our main goal is to explore the heterogeneity of delusions. In the second section, we look at definitions of delusions. The concept of "delusion" can be very elusive, given the difficulty in establishing the necessary and sufficient conditions that a belief must meet to count as a delusion. In the third section, we focus on the clinical characteristics of delusions. Clinically, delusions differ both in form and content, and can be found in the context of a number of mental disorders. In the fourth section, we discuss how clinical delusions share some features with everyday beliefs—which suggests that there is a sense of "delusions" that cuts across the clinical and non-clinical divide. That is the sense of delusions that focuses on its epistemic features.

Clinically, the phenomenon of delusion is truly transdiagnostic, and a variety of methodological approaches, utilising the resources of neuroscience, psychoanalysis, cognitive psychology, and phenomenology, can be adopted in studying it. The term "delusion" is also amply used outside clinical contexts—as in the title of Richard Dawkins' book, "The God Delusion", or the tendency to describe alien abduction beliefs, climate change denialism, and COVID-19 conspiracy theories as delusional. This prompts interesting questions about delusions across and beyond diagnoses. How can we tell delusional beliefs apart from other beliefs? To what extent can delusions be a meaningful response to an uncertain world or to adverse experiences? Are delusions always irrational and pathological beliefs? An integrationist approach that borrows resources and methods from different traditions of thought is well placed to answer those questions and investigate further the nature of delusions, if indeed there is something in common among all the phenomena that attract the label of "delusion".

DOI: 10.4324/9781003288992-15

Defining Features of Delusions

In English-language dictionaries, "delusion" is usually defined as something that is believed to be true or real but that is actually false or unreal. A key feature of delusion is the inability of the person with the delusion to distinguish between what is real and what only seems to be real, often as a result of a pathological or disturbed state of mind (see e.g., Cambridge Dictionary 2022, or Merriam-Webster 2022).

When examined through a clinical lens, various conceptualisations of delusions have been proposed for the purposes of definition and classification, starting from the work of Emil Kraepelin, who first classified mental disorders. In his *Textbook of Psychopathology*, Kraepelin analyzes delusional ideas in his patients and considers delusion as a pathological erroneous belief that cannot be corrected by logical proof to the contrary. Karl Jaspers (1913) offers a more specific characterisation of delusions in his *General Psychopathology*, indicating that delusions, as "the basic characteristic of madness", are disorders of thought. To be a delusion, a belief needs to meet three main criteria: (*a*) to be held with strong subjective certainty, namely with unusual conviction; (*b*) to be incorrigible in front of logic demonstration of the impossibility of the conviction; and (*c*) to have impossible or false content. Also, Jaspers distinguishes delusions in terms of their formal characteristics: *primary delusions* are not understandable, and amount to a "transformation in our total awareness of reality", like delusions in schizophrenia, whereas *delusion-like ideas* are understandable given the patient's psychological status, like delusions in major depression.

Following Kraepelin's and Jaspers' teaching, other psychopathologists have put forward definitions of delusions that substantially share a similar conceptualization of the phenomenon. For example, M.J. Hamilton (1978) underlines that delusions are false, unshakeable beliefs arising from morbid mental processes, and Andrew Sims (1995) defines delusions as false beliefs based on incorrect inference about, or examination of, external reality, firmly sustained despite (almost) everybody else rejecting the beliefs. There is some consensus on delusion being a condition in which: (*a*) a person expresses an idea or belief with unusual persistence or force, even when evidence suggests the contrary; (*b*) this idea or belief appears to have an undue influence on the person's life, and the way of life is often altered to an inexplicable extent; (*c*) any attempt to contradict the idea or belief is likely to arouse an inappropriately strong emotional reaction, often characterised by irritability and hostility; (*d*) the belief content is unlikely to be true, and out of keeping with the individual's social, cultural, and religious background; (*e*) the belief, if acted out, often leads to behaviours which are abnormal, and out of character (even if sometimes those behaviours are understandable in light of the delusional beliefs); (*f*) other people who know the person with the delusion observe that the person's belief and behaviour are uncharacteristic and alien (Munro, 2009).

These conceptualizations of delusion are partially reflected in the American Psychiatric Association's (APA) *Diagnostic and Statistical Manual of Mental Disorders* (DSM-5TR, 2022), and in the World Health Organization's (WHO) *International Classification of Diseases* (ICD-11, 2019). Delusion is "a false belief based on incorrect inference about external reality that is firmly sustained despite what almost everybody else believes and despite what constitutes incontrovertible and obvious proof or evidence to the contrary". A clause is added: "The belief is not one ordinarily accepted by other members of the person's culture or subculture (e.g., it is not an article of religious faith)" (see DSM-5TR, pp. 421–423). Despite the apparent agreement on how to define delusions in the psychiatric literature, offering criteria for delusions is a much more complex and challenging task than it might seem. Whereas some authors broadly agree with Jaspers on how to characterise delusions (see, e.g., Jones et al., 2003), other authors argue that it is difficult if not impossible to define what delusions are (see, e.g., Garety, 1985; David, 1999).

One of the problems in defining delusions is that we expect the distinctions used in psychiatric nosology to be categorical. But determining whether a belief is true or false is not always an easy thing to do, especially considering that some delusional beliefs are *about the external world* (a delusional experience of an object, supported or not by delusional perception, as in "Those people are spies following me to kill me"; "I am sure there are microphones in the room that will transmit my thoughts to Mars"); and other delusional beliefs are *about a person's inner world* (a person's experience of themselves, as in "There is a mass growing inside myself that will explode soon"). Even if we could always establish whether a belief is true or false based on a shared understanding of reality, it is not at all obvious that all delusions are false. Some openly reject falsity as a criterion for delusions and point to other criteria as the key criteria, such as the fact that the person has limited evidence, or no evidence, for the belief (Coltheart, 2007); or the fact that the belief is maintained even when evidence emerges against it (Davies et al., 2001). In such accounts, falsity is not necessary for a belief to be delusional. Rather, what makes a belief delusional is its relationship with evidence. As Vaughan Bell writes, "just because they're out to get you doesn't prove you're not paranoid" (Bell, 2013).

Maybe then incorrigibility captures best what is distinctive about delusions, as it points to how the delusion does not change in the face of counterevidence. It is not uncommon for people to have incorrigible beliefs without being delusional (e.g., Spitzer, 1990; Leeser and O'Donohue, 1999; Feyaerts et al., 2021), so incorrigibility cannot be a sufficient condition for delusions. But can it be a promising necessary condition for it? Incorrigibility is a very demanding notion: if we concede that delusions are *incorrigible*, we are saying that they *cannot change* in the light of evidence or argument. This criterion makes the definition of delusion vulnerable to counterexamples. Admittedly, it is a rare phenomenon to talk someone out of a delusion because the person with the delusion often acknowledges that their belief is being challenged, but then elaborates the belief or dismisses the objection to neutralise the challenge. So, it would seem that some change can occur in how the content is believed, or in the content of the belief itself, but the change does not amount to a correction. That is why some authors prefer not to describe delusions as incorrigible or fixed, but as very resistant to counterevidence: the possibility of change cannot be entirely ruled out, but delusional beliefs are less likely to be abandoned in the face of counterevidence than other beliefs.

One criterion in Munro's list is that the belief is not in keeping with the person's social, cultural, or religious background, and another is that it gives rise to behaviour that is uncharacteristic of that person. But attention to how people describe their experiences prior to the development of the delusion and to people's attitudes towards their delusional realities sometimes tells a different story. The content of the delusion is typically false and often bizarre, and the person may not have evidence for the delusional belief that other people accept as good evidence. But despite its implausibility and ill-groundedness, the content of delusion can be connected to some of the experiences the person had prior to the adoption of the delusional belief, and in that sense, the delusion can have meaning for the person reporting it (Gunn and Bortolotti 2018; Gunn and Larkin 2020). Moreover, some delusions can be empowering and give the person's life some shape and meaning (Ritunnano and Bortolotti 2022; Ritunnano et al. 2022), being related to something the person cares about or contributing to the person feeling important. So, it is not always true that the delusion is out of character or gives rise to behaviour that appears alien: it may be a response to a very traumatic or disruptive event or may be a way to cope with a reality that is difficult to accept.

To add to the challenge of providing criteria for delusions, the high subjective certainty of delusional beliefs, the rigidity of the beliefs, and their resistance to change have all been questioned by recent work in computational psychiatry (e.g., Ashinoff et al. 2022). This research supports the need to have a broader approach to delusions, encompassing both their phenomenological and neurocognitive aspects (Sass and Byrom 2015).

Clinical Characteristics of Delusions

To make the definition problem even more complex is the fact that, from a clinical point of view, psychiatric nosography (DSM-5-TR, ICD-11) indicates the existence of different types of delusions (Coltheart 2013), where distinctions can be made on the basis of how the delusion impacts one's sense of self (see Table 11.1), what formal features the delusion has (see Table 11.2), and what its main theme is (see Table 11.3). Another element

Table 11.1 Delusions and the Self

Delusions and the Self	
CONTROL	Belief that another person, group of people, or external force controls one's general thoughts, feelings, impulses, or behaviours.
THOUGHT BROADCASTING	Belief that one's thought is projected and perceived by others.
THOUGHT INSERTION	Belief that one's thought is not one's own but inserted into one's mind by an external source or entity.
THOUGHT WITHDRAWAL	Belief that one's thoughts have been removed by some outside forces or malicious people.
REFERENTIAL	Belief that insignificant remarks, gestures, comments, environmental cues, etc., are directed at oneself and only oneself, with a related personal meaning or significance.

Table 11.2 Delusional Themes

Themes in Delusional Disorders	
PERSECUTION	Belief of delusional proportion that other people are dangerous and can be harmful.
INFIDELITY	Belief that one's own partner is unfaithful and has an affair with another person).
LOVE	Belief that there is someone, usually a celebrity, in love with oneself.
RELIGION	Belief that one is a god, has god-like powers, or was chosen by a supreme entity to act as a god.
POWER	Belief that one is a celebrity, or more important than other people.
SOMATIC	Belief about one's bodily functioning or sensations, or physical appearance.
GUILT/ UNWORTHINESS	Beliefs related to one's feelings of guilt or sin, or self-accusation of delusional intensity.
NEGATION/ NIHILISTIC	Belief that one does not exist or that one has died, that one has lost one's internal organs, or parts of one's body; belief that one is financially incapacitated.

Table 11.3 Features of Delusions

Features of Delusions	
BIZARRE	Implausible, not understandable, not deriving from ordinary life experiences (e.g., the belief that one has microparticles in one's teeth put by an alien).
NON-BIZARRE	Can be possible, but it is highly unlikely to be true (e.g., the belief that one is controlled by spies who are recording one's conversations).
MOOD-CONGRUENT	Coherent with one's feelings (e.g., a person with depression believes that the news anchors on television highly disapprove of them, or a person in a manic state believes to be a god).
MOOD NEUTRAL	Not related to any emotional state (e.g., the belief that one has worms in one's skin).
MONOTHEMATIC	Circumscribed and isolated from the rest of one's beliefs.
POLYTHEMATIC	Elaborated and integrated with the rest of one's beliefs.

of heterogeneity is that delusions can vary with respect to their severity. The features involved in determining the level of severity of delusional beliefs include: (*a*) the degree to which the person is convinced of the reality of the belief (*conviction of the delusion*); (*b*) the degree to which the belief is close or far from consensual reality according to the person's own culture (*bizarreness of the delusion*); (*c*) the degree to which the belief is systematized, logical, and consistent (*organization or disorganization of the delusion*); (*d*) the degree to which the belief involves an emotional response (*affective implication of the delusion*); (*e*) the degree to which the belief impacts one or more area of the person's life (*extension of the delusion*); (*f*) the degree to which the belief causes preoccupation and concerns in the person (*pressure of the delusion*); and (*g*) the degree to which the person behaviourally acts as a consequence of the belief (*deviant behaviour resulting from delusions*) (see Kendler et al. 1983).

Lastly, when examining the psychiatric disorders in the context of which delusions emerge, we find an extreme heterogeneity of clinical conditions. Delusional beliefs are in fact transdiagnostic and can be symptoms of different disorders (psychotic disorders) or can be a syndrome by themselves (delusional disorders) (Bebbington and Freeman 2017). Delusions can be one of the constellations of symptoms in *schizophrenia spectrum disorders*, which include a variety of different disturbances having psychotic symptoms (mainly diminished or distorted sense of reality, delusions, hallucinations) as one (but not only) of the main characteristics: more precisely schizophrenia, schizoaffective disorder, schizophreniform disorder, and brief psychotic disorder. In all these disorders, delusions are part of a more complex series of clusters of symptoms.

In brief psychotic disorder, alongside with delusions, the patient shows hallucinations, disorganized speech (e.g., derailment, incoherence), and grossly disorganized or catatonic behaviour with a duration of less than one month. Likewise, in schizophreniform disorder, hallucinations, disorganized speech, and grossly disorganized or catatonic behaviour are associated with negative symptoms (i.e., diminished emotional expression, diminished motivation, avolition) with a duration of less than six months (therefore it is a provisional diagnosis). Schizophrenia is characterized by the same symptoms as above, plus by a lowered level of functioning in one or more major areas (e.g., work, interpersonal relations, self-care) for at least six months. In schizoaffective disorder, delusions, hallucinations, disorganized speech, grossly disorganized or catatonic behaviour, and negative symptoms are associated with the symptoms of a major mood episode (major depressive or manic).

So-called *delusional disorders* are clinical conditions in which delusions are the main clinical characteristic. Basically, delusions have a powerful logical construction and internal consistency, do not interfere with general logical reasoning or with disturbance of behaviour (unless when related to the delusional belief system), and are stable over time, making the illness itself a chronic disorder. In delusional disorders the content of the belief can involve erotomania (i.e., the theme of the delusional belief is that one is the object of another person's love); grandiosity (i.e., the theme of the delusion is the conviction that one has some great but unrecognized talent or powers); jealousy (i.e., the theme of the delusion is an unshakeable conviction that one's partner is unfaithful); persecution (i.e., the theme of the delusion is centred on the fact that one is spied, cheated, followed, poisoned, maliciously maligned, and so on); and preoccupation with the body (i.e., the theme of the delusion is that there is something concerning with one's body, mostly bodily changes or organ functions).

Delusions can also be part of *mood disorders*. Both bipolar and major depressive disorders may present psychotic features, which are usually mood-congruent, that is, aligned to the person's mood. For instance, a person with a severe major depressive episode (low mood) can have a nihilistic delusion, and a person in a manic psychotic state can have a grandiose delusion. It is also possible that delusional beliefs are part of a major depressive or manic episode with psychotic features, but mood-incongruent (e.g., persecutory delusion in a depressed patient).

Delusions can also be found in *psychiatric disorders secondary to brain-related alterations*, such as in neurocognitive disorders (mainly delirium and dementia), substance-induced psychotic disorder, or delusion due to a medical disorder. In delirium, disorganized delusions can accompany a series of symptoms indicating an acute state of confusion (e.g., reduced ability to direct, focus, sustain, and shift attention; reduced awareness of the environment; memory deficit, disorientation, alterations in language, visuospatial ability, or perception). When present in dementia, delusions are associated with the main features of the major cognitive disorder such as significant cognitive decline from a previous level of performance in complex attention, executive function, learning and memory, language, perceptual-motor or social cognition. In substance-induced psychotic disorder, the patient's history, physical examination, or laboratory findings clearly indicate the onset of delusions (and hallucinations) temporally after substance intoxication or withdrawal (e.g., amphetamine-type substance, cocaine, cannabis) or after exposure to or withdrawal from a medication, which are therefore identified as the cause of delusion. The patient's history, physical examination, or laboratory findings clearly indicate the onset of delusions (and hallucinations) secondary to somatic disorders (e.g., Cushing's syndrome, brain tumour) that cause delusions.

Delusions beyond the Clinical Context

When we describe a person's belief as delusional, we do not always imply that the belief is symptomatic of a mental disorder. The beliefs we may call "everyday delusions" share some of the features of clinical delusions that we reviewed in the second section but are not typically idiosyncratic to one person and can be shared by groups of people, often well-defined social groups whose views depart from those widely accepted in mainstream society. Beliefs that have been compared to clinical delusions in this respect are COVID-19 denialism and COVID-19 conspiracy beliefs. Denialisms and conspiracy beliefs with different themes (e.g., those centred on climate change) have also been described as delusional on the ground that they are resistant to counterevidence and either implausible in their own right or less plausible than the mainstream beliefs about those phenomena.

Unusual beliefs such as alien abduction beliefs are not considered pathological but share many features with clinical delusions – they are held with high subjective conviction, are resistant to counterevidence, can be distressing, and have a content that is remote from everyday life experience (Sullivan-Bissett 2020). Some people claim that they have been abducted by aliens for the purpose of being examined or experimented upon. This is probably due to their experiencing awareness during sleep paralysis: they feel that their bodies cannot move due to the effect of REM sleep and may have illusory perceptions of breathing with difficulty, flying, floating, and of there being someone in the room (Kinne and Bhanot 2008). If people who have those hallucinations are open to the possibility of alien life, they may interpret their unusual experiences in the light of alien abduction narratives.

Self-evaluations and predictions of one's future that are more positive than is warranted by the evidence at one's disposal have also been compared with delusions for being detached from (and not always constrained by) reality. The nonclinical population is extremely vulnerable to optimistically biased beliefs, and seems to gain from them, to the point that the tendency to adopt those beliefs has been described as adaptive even if the beliefs fail to meet standards of truth or rationality. The phenomenon of *unrealistic optimism* (Jefferson et al. 2017) shows that people without a psychiatric diagnosis can also embrace implausible beliefs and fail to revise them when counterevidence emerges. This optimism can be due to a variety of "positive illusions" (Taylor 1989). In the illusion of control, people believe that they have more power to control external events than is the case. In the superiority illusion, people overestimate their own skills, talents, and virtues. The optimism bias makes people believe that they are less subject to adverse events (such as contracting a serious disease or experiencing a break-up) than the average. Similar to clinical delusions, optimistic beliefs are not easily modified when negative feedback is received—people typically reinterpret negative feedback in a more positive light to maintain a good concept of themselves. Just like clinical delusions, optimistically biased beliefs are often implausible and ill-grounded. However, different from clinical delusions, most optimistically biased beliefs tend to have beneficial effects on people's agency, increasing motivation, pro-social behaviour, and productivity.

The map of similarities and dissimilarities between types of clinical delusions we reviewed in the third section, and the partial overlap between clinical and everyday beliefs we examined here suggest that to further investigate the nature of delusions we may need to combine a number of disciplinary and methodological frameworks (Table 11.4). Some of the frameworks that have been applied to the study of clinical delusions are presented as competitors, whereas others have been fruitfully combined (see Broome and Bortolotti 2009). The psychoanalytic approach according to which delusions are a projection of a person's internal conflict on the external world badly matches the now more influential neurobiological and cognitive psychological approaches according to which delusions are the outcome of some dysfunction in the way in which the brain processes information. However, for some delusions, such as anosognosia (i.e., the denial of an illness or impairment), motivational and cognitive factors are combined to arrive to a satisfactory causal explanation of how the beliefs are formed (Aimola Davies et al. 2009). Similarly, beliefs in conspiracy theories seem to involve both certain biased ways of processing information (such as the intentionality bias where people prefer explanations of negative events involving a person or group deliberately planning those events to cause harm); and motivational factors, such as the need to feel

Table 11.4 Accounts of Delusions

Accounts of Delusions	
NEUROBIOLOGICAL	"Delusion" indicates a series of events having a neurobiological basis that can be explained by empirical neuroscientific research.
PHENOMENOLOGICAL	"Delusion" indicates a person's subjective experience to be studied by psychopathology, without dismissing other scientific approaches.
PSYCHOANALYTIC	"Delusion" indicates the result of a conflict (e.g., latent homosexual tendencies, lack of self-confidence, identity disturbance) between id, ego, and super-ego, with the conflict projected outwards and attributed to the external world.
COGNITIVE-PSYCHOLOGICAL	"Delusion" indicates the output of belief-formation and belief-maintenance processes characterised by anomalous experiential input, a cognitive dysfunction, or a (set of) cognitive biases.
EPISTEMIC	"Delusion" indicates a belief with certain epistemic features, including implausibility, ill-groundedness, unshakeability, and centrality to one's mental life.

in-the-know and in control when a threatening event occurs (such as the need for closure and the need for uniqueness).

The epistemic approach considers the surface features of delusions, that is, how people with delusions tend to behave, and focuses on behaviour that can be captured by using epistemic notions such as those of belief, falsity, evidence, inference, incorrigibility, fixity, and so on. It does not directly address the causal factors responsible for the formation and maintenance of delusional beliefs so it can apply across diagnoses, and also beyond diagnoses. It is via this epistemic approach that we can make sense of the partial overlap between delusions in the clinic and elsewhere; independent of the diagnoses that people attract and the themes of their beliefs, the beliefs themselves share some common features: despite other people finding the beliefs implausible, people hang onto their beliefs to the point that the beliefs may seem unshakeable, and the beliefs tend to play a central role in people's mental life.

Conclusions

What lessons can we draw from the heterogeneity of delusions and the applicability of the term 'delusion' to an increasing number of clinical and nonclinical phenomena? As with all beliefs and experiences reflecting at the same time the person's perspective on the world and the world's influences on the person's behaviour, the study of delusions may benefit from a pluralistic approach, integrating insight from neuroscience, cognitive psychology, psychoanalysis, philosophy, and phenomenology.

We should remain open to the possibility that one approach may shed light on a particular aspect of the phenomenon of delusions without being able on its own to offer a comprehensive account of what delusions are, how they emerge, and why they persist. We should also remember that some apparently incompatible approaches may aim at explaining the same phenomenon, for example, the unshakeability of delusional beliefs, at different levels of explanation, ranging from the subpersonal mechanisms of predictive coding to the personal and social practice of basing belief reports on reasons and evidence.

Similar to Dan Stein's recent defence of an integrative approach to psychiatry (Stein 2021), we can adopt a pragmatic attitude, exploring further all the approaches that give useful insights into delusions, both in clinical practice and in our everyday mutual interactions. This might mean that we should not aim to develop a perfectly coherent and unified account of delusions but, in this journey of exploration, let people's experiences guide new empirical investigations and constrain emerging theories.

References

Aimola Davies AM, Davies M, Ogden JA, Smithson M, White RC. Cognitive and Motivational Factors in Anosognosia. In T Bayne, J Fernàndez (Eds.), *Delusions and Self-Deception: Affective Influences on Belief-Formation*. Hove: Psychology Press, pp. 187–225, 2009.

American Psychiatric Association. *Diagnostic and Statistical Manual of Mental Disorders (DSM-5-TR)*. Washington, DC: American Psychiatric Publishing, 2022.

Ashinoff BK, Singletary NM, Baker SC, Horga G. Rethinking delusions: A selective review of delusion research through a computational lens. *Schizophrenia Research* 2022 Jul;245:23–41.

Bebbington P, Freeman D. Transdiagnostic extension of delusions: schizophrenia and beyond. *Schizophrenia Bulletin* 2017;43:273–282.

Bell V. You needn't be wrong to be called delusional. *The Guardian* 4 August, 2013. https://www.theguardian.com/science/2013/aug/04/truly-madly-deeply-delusional.

Broome M, Bortolotti L (eds.) *Psychiatry as Cognitive Neuroscience: Philosophical Perspectives*. Oxford: Oxford University Press, 2009.

Coltheart M. Cognitive neuropsychiatry and delusional belief. *The Quarterly Journal of Experimental Psychology* 2007;60(8):1041–1062. doi: 10.1080/17470210701338071.

Davies M, Coltheart M, Langdon R, Breen N. Monothematic delusions: Towards a two-factor account. *Philosophy, Psychiatry, and Psychology* 2001;8–2: 133–158.

Cambridge Dictionary. Delusion. Cambridge University Press, 2022. Accessed 15 October, 2022, at: https://dictionary.cambridge.org/dictionary/english/delusion

Merriam-Webster.com Dictionary. Delusion. Merriam-Webster. Accessed 15 October, 2022, at: https://www.merriam-webster.com/dictionary/delusion

Coltheart M. On the Distinction between monothematic and polythematic delusions. *Mind & Language* 2013;28(1):103–112.

David AS. On the impossibility of defining delusions. *Philosophy, Psychiatry, and Psychology* 1999;6:17–20.

Feyaerts J, Henriksen MG, Vanheule S, Myin-Germeys I, Sass LA. Delusions beyond beliefs: a critical overview of diagnostic, aetiological, and therapeutic schizophrenia research from a clinical-phenomenological perspective. *Lancet Psychiatry* Mar 2021;8(3):237–249.

Garety P. Delusions: Problems in definition and measurement. *The British Journal of Medical Psychology* 1985;58:25–34.

Gunn R, Bortolotti L. Can delusions play a protective role? *Phenomenology and the Cognitive Sciences* 2018;17(4):813–833. DOI 10.1007/s11097-017-9555-6.

Gunn R, Larkin M. Delusion formation as an inevitable consequence of a radical alteration in lived experience. *Psychosis* 2020;12(2):151–161.

Hamilton M. *Fish's Outline of Psychiatry* (3rd edition). Bristol: John Wright, 1978.

Kinne P, Bhanot V. I've been abducted by aliens. *Current Psychiatry* 2008;7(7):82.

Jaspers K. *Allgemeine Psychopathologie*, Berlin: Springer, 1913. English translation of the 7th edition: *General Psychopathology*, Baltimore: Johns Hopkins University Press, 1997.

Jefferson A, Bortolotti L, Kuzmanovic B. What is unrealistic optimism? *Consciousness and Cognition: An International Journal* 2017;50:3–11. 10.1016/j.concog.2016.10.005

Jones H, Delespaul P, van Os J. Jaspers was right after all – delusions are distinct form normal beliefs. *The British Journal of Psychiatry* 2003;183:285–286.

Kendler KS, Glazer WM, Morgenstern H. Dimensions of delusional experience. *The American Journal of Psychiatry* 1983;140(4):466–469.

Leeser J, O'Donohue W. What is a delusion? Epistemological dimensions. *Journal of Abnormal Psychology* 1999;108:687–694.

Munro A. *Delusional Disorder: Paranoia and Related Illnesses*. Cambridge, UK: Cambridge University Press, 2009.

Ritunnano R, Bortolotti L. Do delusions have and give meaning? *Phenomenology and the Cognitive Sciences* 2022;21(4):949–968.

Ritunnano R, Kleinman J, Whyte Oshodi D, Michail M, Nelson B, Humpston CS, Broome MR. Subjective experience and meaning of delusions in psychosis: A systematic review and qualitative evidence synthesis. *Lancet Psychiatry* 2022 Jun;9(6):458–476.

Sass L, Byrom G. Phenomenological and neurocognitive perspectives on delusions: A critical overview. *World Psychiatry* 2015;14:164–173.

Sims Andrew. *Symptoms in the Mind: An Introduction to Descriptive Psychopathology*, 2nd edition. London: Saunders, 1995.

Spitzer M. On defining delusions. *Comprehensive Psychiatry* 1990;31:377–397.

Stein D. *Problems of Living*. Rio de Janeiro: Elsevier, 2021.

Sullivan-Bissett E. Unimpaired abduction to alien abduction: Lessons on delusion formation. *Philosophical Psychology* 2020;33(5):679–704.
Taylor SE. *Positive Illusions: Creative Self-Deception and the Healthy Mind.* New York: Basic Books, 1989.
World Health Organization (WHO). *International Classification of Diseases*, 11th edition (ICD.11). Geneva: WHO, 2019.

Index

Printed in Dunstable, United Kingdom

77120475R10127